DIABETES

**Questions
you
have
...Answers
you
need**

Other Books From The People's Medical Society

Take This Book to the Hospital With You

How to Evaluate and Select a Nursing Home

Medicine on Trial

Medicare Made Easy

Your Medical Rights

Getting the Most for Your Medical Dollar

Take This Book to the Gynecologist With You

Take This Book to the Obstetrician With You

Healthy Body Book: Test Yourself for Maximum Health

Blood Pressure: Questions You Have . . . Answers You Need

Your Heart: Questions You Have . . . Answers You Need

The Consumer's Guide to Medical Lingo

150 Ways to Be a Savvy Medical Consumer

Take This Book to the Pediatrician With You

100 Ways to Live to 100

Dial 800 for Health

Your Complete Medical Record

Arthritis: Questions You Have . . . Answers You Need

DIABETES

Questions
you
have
...Answers
you
need

By Paula Brisco

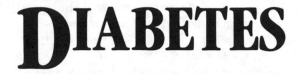
People's Medical Society®

Allentown, Pennsylvania

The People's Medical Society is a nonprofit consumer health organization dedicated to the principles of better, more responsive and less expensive medical care. Organized in 1983, the People's Medical Society puts previously unavailable medical information into the hands of consumers so that they can make informed decisions about their own health care.

Membership in the People's Medical Society is $20 a year and includes a subscription to the *People's Medical Society Newsletter.* For information, write to the People's Medical Society, 462 Walnut Street, Allentown, PA 18102, or call 610-770-1670.

This and other People's Medical Society publications are available for quantity purchase at discount. Contact the People's Medical Society for details.

3 4 5 6 7 8 9 0
First printing, April 1993

CONTENTS

INTRODUCTION

Diabetes is a bad news/good news disease. The bad news is that diabetes is incurable. Medical science has yet to find a cure for one of the world's most common illnesses.

The good news is that diabetes is treatable. With proper medical treatment and a great deal of self-management, most people with diabetes can live a normal length of life with little or no restrictions on their lifestyles.

But the key is treatment—your doctor's and your own. In fact, most of the medical care provided to a person with diabetes is self-care. Unlike many diseases that can be treated only by medical intervention, diabetes is an illness that most can handle quite readily themselves with just a little bit of training from competent medical practitioners.

Diabetes: Questions You Have . . . Answers You Need is your consumer guide to diabetes. Just about every question you could possibly ask is posed in this book, and all of them are answered in detail. You can even find answers to questions you may never have thought of asking.

As the nation's largest consumer health advocacy organization, the People's Medical Society receives tens of thousands of calls and letters each year asking a myriad of questions about health care in general and certain diseases in particular. Diabetes has consistently been one of those conditions.

As we reviewed what was available for the general consumer on the subject, we found that much of what was on the market was either too technical or too oriented to a single approach to diabetes management. We felt that a broader guide, one that answered the questions the People's Medical Society has been asked for more than a decade, would be a valuable addition to consumer medical literature.

Diabetes: Questions You Have . . . Answers You Need is designed to empower you. Utilizing it as an adjunct to medical and self-care can help ensure that diabetes, the disease, does not become diabetes, the centerpiece of your life. That is what empowerment is all about: you having control over your own life.

Longtime People's Medical Society associate Paula Brisco has done a magnificent job of reviewing the medical literature and interviewing experts from a wide range of important fields to put this useful book together. Her skill is her ability to translate the ''medicalese'' into ''consumerese'' to assure you better understanding of this disease.

Diabetes is a serious and dangerous condition. But with knowledge and information, coupled with qualified medical treatment and good self-care, it can be controlled.

Charles B. Inlander
President
People's Medical Society

DIABETES

**Questions
you
have
. . . Answers
you
need**

Terms printed in boldface can be found in the glossary, beginning on page 165. Only the first mention of the word in the text will be boldfaced.

We have tried to use male and female pronouns in an egalitarian manner throughout the book. Any imbalance in usage has been in the interest of readability.

1 THE BASICS

Q: What is diabetes?

A: Diabetes is a malfunction in the body's ability to convert **carbohydrates**—sweet and starchy foods, such as fruit, bread and vegetables—into energy to power the body. The medical name for this is **diabetes mellitus**, meaning "honey-sweet diabetes." As you might gather from such a name, diabetes is characterized by an abnormally high and persistent concentration of sugar in the bloodstream. (Doctors often refer to this as "elevated **plasma glucose**.") Other characteristics are sugar in the urine, excessive urine production and unusual thirst, hunger and weight loss. People affected with diabetes generally require lifelong medical care to control the disease.

Q: Why are carbohydrates a problem?

A: The problem is not so much the carbohydrates per se, but the way the body uses them to create energy. The process of converting food into energy is called **metabolism**, and diabetes is often called a metabolic disorder.

To explain why carbohydrates pose a problem, let's look first at the metabolic system of a healthy person.

In a normal body, carbohydrates are converted to glucose and other simple sugars in the stomach and small intestine. Glucose moves from these organs into the veins. The blood circulates glucose through the body, where it goes to the liver, muscle and fat cells, either to be stored for later use or to be used immediately as energy. Thus, glucose enters body cells, powering the muscles, heart and brain and assisting the body in maintaining a constant temperature.

A body of a person with diabetes also converts carbohydrates to sugars and sends them into the blood. But at this point the system comes to a crashing halt: The glucose is unable to enter the cells.

Q: Why not?

A: The answer has to do with **insulin**, a hormone that enables the body to burn carbohydrates.

Q: Insulin? Where does that come from?

A: It comes from the **pancreas**—a six-inch-long gland that is located behind the stomach. In healthy people, the pancreas secretes many fluids, including insulin.

However, in a person with diabetes, one of two things happens: No insulin—or not enough insulin—is being produced by the pancreas, or what the pancreas does produce is not functioning properly. In either case, the system has gone awry; the end result is that glucose remains in the blood and cannot be processed as energy.

Q: So insulin is important?

A: Absolutely. That one hormone enables the cells to absorb glucose for use as energy. Without it, a "glucose glut" eventually results—high levels of unused blood sugar are trapped in the bloodstream.

Q: How high?

A: Blood-glucose levels vary during the course of the day. In normal adults, blood-glucose levels range between 60 and 100 milligrams per deciliter—designated as mg/dl—of blood plasma when a person is **fasting**. By fasting, the medical profession means that the person hasn't eaten for three or more hours (before breakfast, for example). Blood-glucose numbers are slightly higher for children.

When fasting blood sugar is between 115 and 140 mg/dl, doctors become mildly concerned. If your doctor runs multiple fasting tests on your blood and the results are over 140 mg/dl, you are considered diabetic. In short, your blood-sugar levels are too high.

Q: So what's wrong with high blood sugar?

A: As sugar builds in the bloodstream, the kidneys try to pump it out. To eliminate the sugar, the kidneys must dissolve it. The more sugar there is to be eliminated, the more urine that must be passed.

You can see how this situation quickly leads to frequent urination, increased thirst and dehydration—three of the symptoms of diabetes. Although the kidneys effectively keep the body from becoming overrun with sugar, working double time wears out the kidneys sooner than normal. Over a lifetime, such overwork eventually brings on kidney failure.

But that's not the only problem with high blood sugar.

Q: What's the other?

A: At the same time that the kidneys are furiously flushing the system of sugar, the body is seriously low on fuel. The body's cells, unable to burn sugar, begin to use **protein** and body fat as a source of energy.

This breakdown of fats for fuel releases toxic acids called **ketones**. Some ketones are excreted through the urine. Eventually, however, the ketones accumulate, and at high levels they can lead to a condition called **ketoacidosis**, which is in effect a poisoning of the system. Initial symptoms of this are frequent urination, increased thirst and dry mouth, the latter a result of dehydration. In extreme cases, ketoacidosis can cause unconsciousness—what some people call a **diabetic coma**. If left untreated, ketoacidosis can kill.

Q: So you're saying that diabetes can be life threatening?

A: Definitely. The very nature of the disease puts the sufferer at risk for serious complications. Some experts believe diabetes is now the nation's third or fourth leading cause of death.

Q: What can happen if diabetes goes unchecked?

A: Diabetes hastens wear and tear on many crucial bodily functions. In particular, it attacks:
• The circulatory system. According to the American Diabetes Association, diabetes leads to coronary heart disease, stroke and circulation problems in the hands and feet. These conditions are two to four times more common in people with diabetes, and they account for most of their hospitalizations. Heart attacks, hardening of the arteries, strokes, poor circulation in the feet, amputations—these are concrete and common examples of diabetes damage.
• The kidneys. Diabetes is the leading cause of end-stage kidney disease.
• The eyes. Diabetic eye disease, or diabetic **retinopathy**, is the major cause of new vision loss in Americans 20 to 74 years old, according to the National Eye Institute.
• The nervous system. Nerve cells may be disturbed or damaged, causing severe pain or loss of feeling—a condition known as **neuropathy**.

We examine in detail the complications of diabetes in Chapter 4. For now, it suffices to say that diabetes must be treated seriously. In nearly all situations, people with diabetes require, at a minimum, routine medical treatment—including daily self-care.

Left unchecked, diabetes shortens life. It is not a condition that goes away.

Q: What can be done about it?

A: Quite simply, you must learn to control your diabetes. Don't let it control you! Many people with diabetes have taken personal responsibility for managing their disease and, as a result, they live normal, productive lives. If any disorder can be called a lifestyle disease, diabetes comes as close as any. Just by controlling blood sugar, the severity of diabetic complications can be prevented.

So, the most obvious step is to get blood-sugar levels down to normal. For some people, that means taking insulin; for others, it means losing weight; for some, it means both. For all people with diabetes, it means paying particular attention to diet and exercise—what we mean by a lifestyle change.

All of the experts in the field recount the importance of sound health habits that can help control diabetes and, in some cases, prevent it. You'll find plenty of hands-on information about managing diabetes right here in this book, and we'll guide you to additional resources.

But whatever their lifestyles, the very first steps for all people with diabetes are to find out that they have the disease and to realize that they're not alone.

Q: How many people have diabetes?

A: In the world, probably well over 100 million. In the United States, estimates of the number of people affected by the disease run as high as 14 million—and that number increases each year. That includes people of all ages, from children to the elderly. The American Diabetes Association estimates that 6 percent of the general U.S. population over age 40 has been found to have diabetes—and an equal amount has not been diagnosed yet.

Q: You mean some people have diabetes and don't know it?

A: Approximately 6 million people, according to the American Diabetes Association.

Q: How can that be?

A: Scientists estimate that the onset of the disease can be anywhere from 4 to 12 years. That means someone may have diabetes 5, 8, even 10 years before it's diagnosed, depending upon the kind of diabetes that person has. Unfortunately, in that time the condition can damage the body.

Many folks only find out about their diabetes once they're having trouble with their eyes, nerves, kidneys, blood vessels or heart.

Q: I think you just said that there's more than one kind of diabetes. Is that correct?

A: Yes. Although people tend to think of diabetes as one disease, it really is a group of disorders. What they all have in common is a problem with insulin production or insulin action.

Q: Can you give some examples of the different disorders?

A: Let's start by looking at the two most common, **type-I diabetes** and **type-II diabetes**.

TYPE-I DIABETES

Q: What is this?

A: Type-I diabetes is the most severe form of diabetes. It is also known as **insulin-dependent diabetes**. People with type-I diabetes generally depend on injections of insulin to regulate their sugar metabolism.

In the past, type-I diabetes was called **juvenile diabetes** because doctors thought that it would strike only children or young adults. Doctors now know that people of any age can develop type-I diabetes, although the majority of cases are discovered in people under 20 years of age.

People with type-I diabetes are vulnerable to dangerous short-term complications of the disease. Two of these complications have to do with disruptive swings in blood-sugar levels, such as **hyperglycemia** (too much blood sugar) and **hypoglycemia** (too little blood sugar). People with type-I diabetes also are at particular risk of ketoacidosis—that dangerous buildup of toxic acids in the body that we mentioned earlier.

Q: How many people have type-I diabetes?

A: Almost all Caucasian diabetic children have type I, while about 10 percent of adult diabetics have type I, according to George S. Eisenbarth, M.D., of the Joslin Diabetes Center and Harvard Medical School, in Boston. But even that fraction translates into big numbers: somewhere around 1 million Americans.

Q: What causes it?

A: Experts call type-I diabetes an **autoimmune** disease and suggest that it is genetically programmed. (*Autoimmune* is a term used to describe what happens when the body's immune system attacks itself.) The scenario goes something like this:

Inside the pancreas are approximately 100,000 cell clusters known as the **islets of Langerhans**, or **islets**. (Crossword puzzle buffs are probably very familiar with this term.) Each islet may include 1,000 to 2,000 **beta cells**, which manufacture insulin and release it into the bloodstream when blood-glucose levels rise. In people with type-I diabetes, beta cells are attacked by the immune system and are slowly destroyed. Eventually production of insulin comes to a halt because no beta cells remain.

Scientists are not quite sure what causes the body's immune system to sabotage pancreatic cells, although they have detected a genetic predisposition to this disorder. Many scientists also believe that a trigger, perhaps a virus, must be present to start the destruction.

Q: How long does this destruction take?

A: Probably four to seven years, according to recent research. Unfortunately, symptoms don't arise until 80 to 90 percent of the beta cells are destroyed. Once that happens, sudden and dramatic symptoms appear. The disease is quickly detected and diagnosed at that point.

Q: What are the symptoms?

A: They include frequent urination, constant thirst and hunger and weight loss. Some people have fatigue, blurred vision and recurrent skin infections. Medical tests show elevated blood-sugar levels and sugar in the urine.

Q: Can this form of diabetes be prevented?

A: At present, doctors cannot prevent type-I diabetes. Nor is it something that could have been avoided by those people who have it.

But researchers are busily looking for a way to identify both the predisposing genetic factors and the viral or environmental triggers of the disease. They reason that if they could detect cell destruction early, a method of treatment known as **immunotherapy** could be used to stop the body from destroying the beta cells, thus halting the disease's progression. We talk about new areas of research later in this chapter.

TYPE-II DIABETES

Q: What is meant by type II?

A: Type II is often called **non-insulin-dependent diabetes**. Formerly called **adult-onset diabetes** or **maturity-onset diabetes**, it seldom develops in people under the age of 40. However, experts are quick to point out that age is an unreliable indicator of diabetes type, since a person of any age can develop type-II diabetes. Type-II diabetes in children and adolescents is sometimes called **maturity-onset diabetes of the young** and given the acronym MODY.

Q: How common is type-II diabetes?

A: It accounts for some 85 to 90 percent of all cases of diabetes, and usually shows up in middle-aged to older adults. Four out of five of these people are overweight—and in most cases, these people were overweight *before* their diabetes developed.

To an even greater extent than with type I, type II runs in families. But it's generally thought that a combination of excess weight and age triggers the genetic predisposition.

Q: How else does type-I diabetes differ from type II?

A: A major difference is that people with type-I diabetes must use insulin to live. Their bodies cannot produce this hormone because their beta cells have been irrevocably destroyed. Although some people with type-II diabetes eventually become insulin dependent, most can control their sugar levels through some combination of drugs, weight loss, diet and exercise.

The biggest difference is that people with type-II diabetes, by controlling their disease, are able to reverse the disease process so that insulin is produced and functions normally.

Q: Why is that?

A: People with type-II diabetes still produce the hormone insulin, but it does not function properly. The problem is tied to being overweight. Generally, someone who is chronically obese has a high carbohydrate intake, and that places a strain on his body's glucose metabolism. At the same time, obesity reduces the body's sensitivity to insulin by causing insulin **receptors** on the cells' surfaces to resist insulin. Those cells (primarily muscle and fat cells) then cannot take glucose from the blood, and diabetes results.

In response to the resulting high blood sugar, beta cells in the pancreas struggle to produce more and more insulin. Eventually this overproduction exhausts the beta cells and insulin secretion becomes inadequate.

Q: Is this what is meant by the term **insulin resistance**?

A: Doctors often use that term to indicate that insulin is present but is not being used efficiently. The reason for insulin resistance is not completely understood, although scientists are striving to learn more about it. Recent research suggests that in some cases it may have to do with the way skeletal muscles store glucose for later use. For us, it's enough to know that insulin resistance plays a role in type-II diabetes.

People with type-II diabetes are sometimes given drugs, called **oral hypoglycemic agents**, to increase the secretion and effectiveness of insulin. But there's another way to reverse their problems: by cutting back on food intake and losing weight. Apparently, according to various experts, a weight loss of as little as 10 to 15 pounds can make a difference in the need for medications to control type-II diabetes.

Q: If I can take drugs for type-II diabetes, then why should I worry about my sugar?

A: It's true that in type-II diabetes glucose abnormalities may be mild. But that doesn't mean they are any less dangerous. Again, prolonged hyperglycemia—one of the disorders associated with all types of diabetes—wears on the body and leads to long-term complications.

Q: Is type-II diabetes easy to spot?

A: Actually, no. This form of diabetes is often hard to detect for several reasons.
• The disease typically exhibits no symptoms for many years, and the onset and progression of symptoms can be slow.
• Typical symptoms are not always present.
• Symptoms are mild and may go unnoticed, which helps explain why there may be millions of people who do not know they have diabetes.

Q: What are the symptoms of type-II diabetes?

A: The symptoms of type-II diabetes are similar to those of type I, and include the following: frequent urination, increased thirst, increased hunger, prolonged and unexplained fatigue, blurred vision, numbness or tingling or burning sensations in the legs or feet, slow-healing wounds or sores, gynecological fungal infections in women and sexual impotence in men. All too often, however, the symptoms may be very subtle, or they may imitate another disease. And in some cases no symptoms occur at all. It may take years before symptoms manifest themselves.

Q: **Then how do people find out that they have type II?**

A: Most people find out they have type-II diabetes when a routine blood test unearths high blood-glucose levels or when they visit a doctor to be treated for symptoms of one of the complications of diabetes.

Q: **My doctor isn't sure whether I have type-I diabetes or type II. How can that be?**

A: As you may have noticed, there are many similarities between the symptoms of type-I and type-II diabetes. In the early stages of the disease, it is not always easy to determine which form someone has developed, because some people experience characteristics of both.

Q: **Isn't there some routine test that can distinguish one type from another?**

A: Alas, no quick and easy test exists to distinguish between type I and type II. For many doctors, the road to determining what type of diabetes a patient has is filled with trial and error. It involves trying one treatment approach and, if that doesn't work, trying another.

The consumer's job in such a case is to read up on diabetes, in this book and others, and to work with health-care practitioners in developing and following a treatment plan. The ultimate goal, of course, is to reach and maintain normal blood-sugar levels.

On the other hand, it's possible that you have another form of diabetes.

Q: Besides type I and type II, what other kinds of diabetes are there?

A: There are several other forms of glucose abnormalities, as doctors often call them. Some of these are not diabetes, but they may signal that diabetes is developing. We will look at four: **increased risk for diabetes, impaired glucose tolerance, secondary diabetes** and **gestational diabetes**.

INCREASED RISK FOR DIABETES

Q: How is "increased risk for diabetes" a form of diabetes?

A: Actually, this category is not a form of diabetes per se. But someone who is classified as being in this group may be at increased risk of developing diabetes one day. Think of this as a warning flag, urging the consumer to pay more attention to his or her health.

As described in the *Joslin Diabetes Manual* (12th edition; Philadelphia: Lea & Febiger, 1989), this type of glucose abnormality includes two categories. The first refers to people with **previous abnormality of glucose tolerance** (formerly called *prediabetes*). People with this have no sign of abnormal glucose metabolism, but they experienced a period of impaired glucose tolerance or high blood sugar in the past. Women who have had gestational diabetes are also placed in this group.

The second category is called **potential abnormality of glucose**. People who have a close relative with type-I diabetes or people with islet-cell antibodies are considered part of this group.

Q: How do doctors treat these people?

A: They don't, because there's really nothing to treat. Doctors should monitor the blood-sugar levels of these folks, however, in case something develops down the road.

IMPAIRED GLUCOSE TOLERANCE

Q: Impaired glucose tolerance—that's a strange term. What does it mean?

A: Glucose tolerance is said to be impaired when blood-sugar levels are higher than normal but not high enough to be diagnosed as diabetes. This impairment is indicated by a fasting-blood-glucose reading between 115 and 140 mg/dl. Symptoms of diabetes are generally absent.

Q: How is this condition related to diabetes?

A: Strictly speaking, doctors don't consider impaired glucose tolerance a true form of diabetes, but instead an abnormality in glucose levels—something between normal and "overt diabetes," as the medical profession terms it. A person who has impaired glucose tolerance may improve, so that blood-sugar levels become normal, or may remain unchanged, with sugar levels steady in that gray area between normal and high. Perhaps a quarter of people with impaired glucose tolerance go on to develop diabetes.

Q: Is impaired glucose tolerance dangerous?

A: It doesn't appear that this condition causes severe complications of diabetes, such as kidney failure. But researchers believe that people with impaired glucose tolerance are more likely to have high blood pressure and high **cholesterol** levels—conditions long implicated in coronary heart disease.

SECONDARY DIABETES

Q: What is this?

A: This term is used to describe a host of other conditions that can give rise to diabetes.

Q: Such as?

A: In many such cases, the diabetes is a secondary condition that results from another disease, medication or chemical. Among the causes of secondary diabetes are pancreatic diseases (especially chronic pancreatitis in alcoholics), hormonal abnormalities (including ones that result from the administration of steroids), insulin-receptor disorders, drug- or chemical-induced diabetes and certain genetic syndromes.

Q: You mean to say that drugs can create a form of diabetes?

A: In some instances, yes, because they increase blood sugar to abnormally high levels.

Q: What drugs cause this problem, and is the problem permanent or does it go away when the person stops taking the drug?

A: Certain prescription drugs, including glucocorticoids (used as anti-inflammatories), furosemide (a diuretic, used in blood-pressure control), thiazide diuretics (used in blood-pressure control), estrogen-containing products (such as oral contraceptives and hormone-replacement therapy) and beta blockers (used to treat heart disorders) may produce high blood sugar. Any diagnosis of diabetes should take into account the consumer's history of prescription-drug use.

GESTATIONAL DIABETES

Q: Is this a form of diabetes that affects women?

A: Yes. Gestational diabetes is any type of diabetes that first appears—or is first recognized—during pregnancy. It develops because of the distinctive hormonal environment and metabolic demands of pregnancy. In 95 percent of the cases, the diabetes disappears after childbirth.

For some women (about 5 percent), however, the diabetes remains. And once a woman has had gestational diabetes, she's at risk for developing another form of diabetes (usually type II) later in life.

Q: How many women get gestational diabetes?

A: Approximately 3 percent of pregnant women develop gestational diabetes, but it seems to be more common in women over 25. They account for approximately 50 percent of pregnancies but 85 percent of gestational diabetic pregnancies, according to one medical journal. The risk seems to be similar in first and subsequent pregnancies.

Q: Is it dangerous?

A: Gestational-diabetes symptoms are generally mild and not life threatening to the woman. The condition, however, can pose problems for the infant, including hypoglycemia (low blood sugar) and respiratory-distress syndrome. Women with gestational diabetes are more susceptible than normal to developing **toxemia**, a life-threatening condition for both mother and child.

Q: Is gestational diabetes easy to control?

A: Some women find they need to take insulin, but for the most part, diet and exercise can control gestational diabetes. We talk more about this form of diabetes later in the book.

Q: Back to diabetes in general, can I tell on my own what kind of diabetes I have?

A: Not really—you'd have to work with your doctor to determine that.

The problem with self-diagnosis is that symptoms vary from person to person. And with diabetes, the manner of onset differs from one form to another. In type-I diabetes the manifestations are often abrupt, while in many cases of type-II diabetes the disease has no symptoms. But because the forms of diabetes have so many symptoms in common, you can't make an easy judgment.

Q: Again, in general, those symptoms are . . . ?

A: If you're looking for a rough guideline, here's what the medical literature mentions as important symptoms of untreated or inadequately treated diabetes:

• **Polyuria**: This is the passing of too much urine, or frequent urination.

• Thirst: As you might suspect, polyuria causes dehydration which, in turn, causes thirst.

• Weight loss: The loss of water, as the kidneys strive to eliminate the excess sugar, causes weight loss. Further contributing to weight loss is the need for the body to use protein and fat to supply the energy that normally would be supplied by properly metabolized glucose.

Tiredness is often present in diabetes, but is not considered a sure symptom since it can be associated with many other disorders. Other symptoms include unrelenting hunger, itching of the genitals and skin, visual disturbances (such as blurry vision), skin disorders (for example, boils) and pain and/or numbness of the extremities.

Q: Is there a profile of the typical person with diabetes?

A: If you mean, Is there a one-size-fits-all description? the answer is no. All people are vulnerable to the disease throughout their lives.

Admittedly, statistics point to times of life when diabetes is more likely to occur. As one doctor describes it, "there is a gradual increase in susceptibility, with slight peaks at puberty and during pregnancy, until we reach the age of 40. Then there is a rapid jump." So it's more common to talk about "susceptibility" and the risk factors associated with the disease, rather than what causes it.

Q: What are those risk factors?

A: For starters, the top two are heredity and obesity.

Q: So diabetes can run in families?

A: Yes. Quite simply, if you have a family history of diabetes, especially parents or siblings with diabetes, then you're near the top of the list in terms of risk. Experts term heredity the most important predisposing factor, particularly for type-I diabetes.

Type-II diabetes also tends to run in families, but since 80 to 85 percent of all cases occur among people who are over 40 and overweight, doctors believe obesity is a major player in the development of this form of the disease.

Q: So we're back to the topic of obesity again?

A: That's correct. As we mentioned earlier, 80 to 85 percent of people with type-II diabetes are overweight. True, not all overweight people have diabetes, but they could be setting themselves up for this disease 10 or 20 years hence. As one expert puts it, "events that occur in middle life (excessive weight gain, for example) can have profound clinical effects 20 years later."

Q: What is the definition of "overweight"?

A: To the American Diabetes Association, that means more than 20 percent over ideal body weight.

Q: How about race—is it a risk factor?

A: In the United States the disease is more common among African-Americans, Hispanics and American Indians. In the general population, for example, diabetes-related deaths were 38 per 100,000 people in 1989. For African-Americans, however, diabetes-related mortality was 68 per 100,000 people, and for American Indians/Alaska natives, it was 63 per 100,000.

Scientists stress, however, that race alone does not predict diabetes; it must be combined with another factor, such as obesity.

For example, a recent National Institutes of Health study reported that being African-American isn't an independent risk factor for type-II diabetes. The link between race and diabetes varies according to an individual's weight. At 100 percent desirable weight (meaning as close as possible to ideal weight), African-Americans and Caucasians had the same risk for diabetes. But at 125 percent of desirable weight, the risk in African-Americans was 1.5 times greater than that of Caucasians and was 1.8 greater at 150 percent of desirable weight.

Q: Any other risk factors?

A: Researchers have uncovered a link between poverty and diabetes. Two consumer surveys, conducted by the Gallup Organization in 1989 and in 1990, found a clear relationship between household income and diabetes incidence. In the surveys, households with the lowest income—under $15,000—had by far the highest incidence of the disease.

Q: What else increases susceptibility to diabetes?

A: A few more factors—some that we've already touched on in this chapter—are:
   • Being over age 40 years and having any of the preceding factors
   • Having impaired glucose tolerance
   • Having high blood pressure or high cholesterol levels (240 mg/dl or more)
   • In women, having a history of gestational diabetes or delivery of babies weighing more than 9 pounds

Q: In other words, a person with any one of those risk factors will get diabetes?

A: Not necessarily. For the most part, the presence of one risk factor does not predict diabetes, but it does suggest a possibility. The more risk factors you have, the greater your chance of developing diabetes. According to the American Diabetes Association, the chance of finding diabetes in someone without a risk factor is low.

Q: How is diabetes diagnosed?

A: At one time, diagnosis consisted of taste testing the urine. If it was sweet, that was a confirmation of diabetes mellitus. Fortunately, at least for diagnosticians, things are different today. Diabetes is usually confirmed by the typical signs and symptoms, as well as by high glucose levels in the blood and/or urine. In symptomless people, high blood sugar usually is enough for a diagnosis. On the other hand, it is possible for someone to have some glucose in her urine and not have diabetes, just as it is possible for a person to have mild and moderate elevations in glucose levels but not have diabetes.

When diabetes is suspected, or when a routine blood test reveals high sugar levels (above 200 mg/dl), two simple tests are often performed.

Q: Must I go to my doctor for these tests, or can I use one of those blood-measurement kits in the drugstore?

A: To diagnose diabetes, you should visit your doctor. The kits that you are thinking of can come in handy later if you have diabetes. They are used by people with diabetes to keep track of their day-to-day blood-sugar levels. As a tracking technique, **self-monitoring of blood glucose**, or **SMBG** as the medical profession calls it, plays a crucial role in managing diabetes. It gives the information needed to balance food intake, exercise, and insulin or medication.

Self-testing is an important aspect of self-care, and we talk at great length about it in Chapter 5. But for now, the major diagnostic tests are performed in a doctor's office.

Q: Okay, then, what are the two simple tests that doctors use, and how do they work?

A: The **fasting plasma glucose test** is performed after a person hasn't eaten for 8 to 12 hours, usually first thing in the morning. To diagnose diabetes, several of these tests are given on different days. Glucose levels higher than 140 mg/dl in two successive tests confirm diabetes.

The **oral glucose-tolerance test** begins with a fasting blood sample taken after a person has eaten a high-carbohydrate diet for three days. After that sample is taken, the consumer drinks a glucose solution. Next, blood samples are taken every 30 minutes for two hours, and another sample is taken an hour later. Those blood samples show how the body handles glucose. Normally, blood levels rise after the glucose is drunk and then return to normal. In people with diabetes, blood-sugar levels don't fall that quickly. Blood-glucose levels higher than 200 mg/dl one to two hours after a meal confirm diabetes. If the blood sugar registers over 200 mg/dl after the fasting segment of this test, there's no doubt that the person has diabetes.

Q: **If doctors can do a blood test at any time to confirm diabetes, isn't there any way to detect it earlier?**

A: You've put your finger on an important area of diabetes research. Scientists are looking at both diabetes triggers—factors that spark diabetes onset—and diabetes **markers**—genetic signposts, in a manner of speaking. The idea is that one day, doctors can find those people who will get diabetes and can stop the disease before it starts.

Q: **What do you mean by a trigger?**

A: External environmental factors—such as exposure to a virus, exposure to certain chemicals or nutritional habits—that trigger an inherited, or genetic, predisposition to diabetes. Scientists think many different triggers may be responsible for 70 to 95 percent of type-I cases.

Q: **Are doctors finding these triggers?**

A: Yes. One study, reported in the July 1992 issue of the *New England Journal of Medicine*, points to cow's milk in infants as an environmental trigger of type-I diabetes.

The article notes that "this study strongly suggests that antibodies to albumin in cow's milk also attack the child's own pancreatic beta cells; thus an immunologic reaction to cow's milk may precipitate diabetes in susceptible children." Based on those findings, the American Academy of Pediatrics recommends that parents *do not* give whole cow's milk to infants under a year of age. In addition, some experts postulate that breast-fed infants may be protected against the risk of type-I diabetes later in life.

Q: **I've heard a lot lately about genetic research and testing. Are there any advances taking place in this arena?**

A: Physicians and researchers are making headway in identifying markers—those genetic indications that a person may develop diabetes.

Q: **Such as?**

A: One marker appears to be changes in the way the pancreas secretes insulin. Scientists can use special blood tests to identify, with near certainty among first-degree relatives of people with type-I diabetes, those who will develop diabetes. These *assays*, as the tests are called, identify individuals with insulin or islet-cell antibodies.

More research is under way. According to the *Joslin Diabetes Manual*, other researchers have located two **antigens** (proteins or enzymes capable of stimulating action in the immune system) that serve as markers. These antigens, known as HLA-B8 and HLA-B15, are attacked by the antibodies and white blood cells that make up part of the body's immune system. HLA-B8 and HLA-B15 are more common in people with type-I diabetes than in people without diabetes.

Q: How do researchers use this information?

A: Because scientists have the ability to predict the development of type-I diabetes in some people, investigators have begun to halt or even prevent beta-cell destruction in such individuals.

Q: You mean prevent the destruction even before it starts? How?

A: The most dramatic example comes from a small study in which the onset of type-I diabetes was delayed several years in high-risk children.

Brothers and sisters of kids with diabetes injected themselves with a low dose of insulin each day to improve beta-cell function. All 12 children in the study had normal glucose-tolerance tests at the outset. But over the next few years, those at high risk were identified based on specific tests.

"Our study showed that it is possible to predict who is going to get diabetes among high-risk relatives, and that it is possible to introduce interventions so that we can begin to postpone, delay or even prevent diabetes altogether," says Richard Keller, M.D., one of the study's authors.

Q: Have there been other inroads?

A: Researchers have found that a pancreatic enzyme known as "64K" stimulates production of antibodies in the blood of many people who eventually develop diabetes. It is not yet clear whether the antibodies play a direct role in destroying insulin-producing cells or whether they are a secondary effect of an autoimmune attack by other cells. In any case, researchers believe they are a sign of impending diabetes. And because this enzyme is the same as an enzyme present in large quantities in the brain, researchers expect that the finding may lead to a simple test to screen for people who are likely to develop the disease years before symptoms appear.

Q: Hold on a minute—while this new research is wonderful for the prevention of diabetes, what about those of us who already have diabetes?

A: Doctors are looking into ways to replace beta cells in the pancreas, primarily through transplantation.

Q: Transplantation? You mean surgery that treats diabetes?

A: For some people, yes. Today, pancreas transplantation is the only way for people with type-I diabetes to go off insulin. When the pancreas is replaced, the body once again has enough functioning beta cells to produce insulin. The success of pancreas transplants, however, is fairly limited. In 1992, whole pancreas transplants had a one-year success rate of about 70 percent and a five-year success rate of about 50 percent.

Q: Can anyone receive a new pancreas?

A: Doctors are currently very selective about pancreatic transplantation. Organ rejection remains a major problem—if the organ you receive does not match your own tissues closely enough, your immune system will attack it. **Immunosuppressive drugs** help protect the new organ and weaken the rejection response, but they are risky.

Because of the risks of the immunosuppressive drugs required for transplantation, many surgeons transplant pancreases only in patients with type-I diabetes and only when their kidneys have begun to fail. The pancreas is transplanted along with a kidney.

Anyone interested in pancreatic transplantation should thoroughly discuss the pros and cons with his health-care practitioner. A hefty price tag comes with the operation— close to $100,000 in 1992. On top of that are what doctors call "maintenance" costs of about $10,000 a year. As always, it's best to find a hospital and a surgeon who have plenty of experience with this precise type of surgery. One such place is the Mayo Clinic in Rochester, Minnesota; another is the Joslin Diabetes Center, in Boston.

Q: Will a successful pancreas transplant stop the development of diabetic complications?

A: The medical profession is still debating this. Some doctors are enthusiastic. A report from Sweden indicates that kidney disease does not come back in patients who receive both a kidney and pancreas transplant, and German researchers report that progression of diabetic eye disease slowed and circulation in the small blood vessels of the legs and feet improved after pancreas transplantation.

Other doctors point out that some complications may already have set in by the time a transplant is indicated, and that the complications will continue despite the new pancreas.

Q: This matter of who is eligible for a transplant and who does the best is confusing. Where can I go for more information?

A: If you're interested in transplantation, we suggest you go to your local hospital library and do some research in the medical journals. Then talk to your doctor.

In addition, the American Diabetes Association can update consumers on transplantation and where it is being done (see the Resources section at the end of Chapter 5).

Q: What if I'm not eligible for a pancreas transplant or don't want one. Is any other form of surgery available?

A: Two other surgical treatments are currently under investigation:

• Transplantation of parts of the pancreas—the islets, which contain the beta cells that manufacture insulin. Transplanting the islets makes a person insulin independent for at least several years, according to an article in the *Journal of the American Medical Association*. However, cell rejection is still a problem, and so this surgery is still only experimental. Those people who have islet-cell transplants are part of research studies.

- A less-invasive method of restoring beta cells is also under investigation. Researchers at the University of Wisconsin have been transplanting beta cells, obtained from the pancreas of an adult or a fetus, in people undergoing kidney transplants. Again, cell rejection is a problem with this approach, as is true of any organ replacement.

Q: What about using an artificial pancreas?

A: You may have heard about the device invented by a physician at Tufts University School of Medicine in Boston. He calls his artificial pancreas an ultrafiltering hybrid organ, and he claims the device shields the beta cells of the pancreas from attack by white blood cells. This device has not been tested, so results of its use—positive or negative—are many years down the road.

But as things stand now, most people with diabetes do not expect a transplant. Diabetes is something they learn to live with.

Q: In effect, you're saying that diabetes is a lifelong disease.

A: For most people, yes. In cases of gestational diabetes, women may find that normal sugar levels reappear. Other people with diabetes—those with type II—may be fortunate and find that controlling their weight also controls their blood sugar. For most people, however, having diabetes means making a lifelong commitment to understanding and paying careful attention to what they eat and how they exercise. We talk about these points in the next chapters.

2 INSULIN AND TYPE-I DIABETES

Q: Insulin and type-I diabetes—do the two always go together?

A: Eventually, yes. As we explained in Chapter 1, type-I diabetes is also known as insulin-dependent diabetes. People with type-I diabetes lose the ability to manufacture the hormone insulin. Thus, they need to receive insulin, most frequently in the form of injections, to regulate the way their bodies use food for energy.

Some people who are diagnosed as having type-I diabetes do not immediately require insulin, because their bodies continue to produce small amounts of that hormone. As the disease progresses, however, insulin production stops, and injections are necessary.

Q: Do people with type-II diabetes take insulin?

A: Most people with type-II diabetes are able to control their blood-sugar levels through some combination of drugs, weight loss, diet and exercise. That's why they are also called non-insulin dependent.

However, some become insulin dependent—sometimes intermittently, sometimes for life. In those cases, much of what we talk about in this chapter applies to them, as well.

Q: Can insulin injections cure diabetes?

A: Not by a long shot. (Pardon the pun.) Insulin injections merely compensate for the hormone's absence from the body. They modify the symptoms of the disease but they don't treat the cause. "Time in a bottle" is how the American Diabetes Association describes insulin's effectiveness.

In a most basic sense, insulin controls diabetes that cannot be controlled by diet alone. Insulin works in *conjunction* with a disciplined approach to diet—it is not a replacement for diet. If people with diabetes are not careful about the foods they eat and when they eat those foods, they will not be able to control their blood-sugar levels, regardless of insulin intake.

Although this chapter focuses on the role of insulin and how people use it, the fact is that people with type-I diabetes need both insulin injections and regimented diets to live. Diet is such an important issue for all people with diabetes that we've devoted the lion's share of Chapter 5 to that topic.

Q: You've mentioned the words "discipline" and "regimented" in conjunction with diet. What do you mean?

A: We mean that most people with diabetes who are insulin dependent lead a fairly structured life. Insulin injections (the most common means of putting insulin into the bloodstream—we discuss others later in this chapter), meals and exercise are carefully scheduled. Even the amount of food and exercise are mapped out in advance. All this structure is necessary to keep blood sugar in a normal range—what the medical profession calls **normoglycemia** or **euglycemia**.

You can look at it this way: Controlling blood sugar is like walking a tightrope between too much and too little sugar in the blood. Too much (hyperglycemia) over the years leads to the life-threatening ailments touched on in Chapter 1. Blood-sugar levels that are too low (hypoglycemia) cause irritability, fainting or even death. Eating the right foods, controlling the amount of food you ingest and maintaining the proper amount of insulin in the bloodstream are all essential to keeping your footing on the high wire.

Q: Where does insulin come from?

A: There are several kinds or **species** of insulin. **Beef-derived insulin** is obtained from beef pancreases; **pork-derived insulin** comes from pork pancreases. **Human insulin**, a drug chemically identical to the insulin normally produced by the body, is manufactured in one of two ways: either by using recombinant DNA technology or by chemical modification of pork insulin. The human insulins are known as **synthetic** and **semisynthetic** respectively.

These insulins come in different forms, each of which acts in a different way.

Q: What are those forms?

A: They are short-acting, intermediate-acting and long-acting.

Short-acting insulins go by the names of **regular** and **semilente**. (Short-acting insulins are sometimes referred to as fast-acting insulins, as the word *fast* refers to the speed with which the insulin begins to lower blood-sugar levels.) Short-acting insulins begin acting in about half an hour and their effect lasts approximately one to five hours.

Intermediate-acting insulins come in two forms: **lente** and **NPH**. Preparations with a predetermined proportion of NPH mixed with regular, such as 70 percent NPH to 30 percent regular, are considered intermediate-acting insulins. These begin acting in about 1½ hours and last approximately 12 to 24 hours.

Long-acting insulins include **PZI** (short for protamine zinc insulin) and **ultralente**. These begin to take effect in 4 to 6 hours and can last up to 36 hours.

Q: So which of these forms are most commonly used by people with type-I diabetes?

A: Actually, most people use several forms of insulin. One common approach is to use one form in the

morning and another form later in the day. Other people mix insulin forms in the same syringe because they and their doctors have found that mixtures of short-acting with intermediate- or long-acting insulins do a better job of keeping blood-sugar levels normal than does use of a single insulin alone. But to answer your question, the most commonly used insulins today are regular, semilente, NPH, lente and ultralente.

Because different types of insulin have different pharmacological properties, one form may be preferred over another. According to a report in the journal *Diabetes Care*, human insulin is recommended for women who are pregnant or considering pregnancy, for people who are allergic to animal-derived insulins, for people who are just beginning insulin therapy and for those who must use insulin only intermittently. In fact, most people today are started on human insulin unless they need the long-acting variety, which only comes in beef- or pork-derived forms.

Q: Wait a minute—did I hear you say that a person with diabetes can be allergic to insulin?

A: Yes. He can be allergic to certain types. In particular, beef- and pork-derived insulins, the oldest members of the insulin family, can cause allergic reactions around the spot where the insulin was injected (known as the **injection site**).

Q: What kind of allergic reactions do people get?

A: Reactions can range in intensity from a small, red or itchy area to a widespread skin rash, stomach upset and even difficulty breathing. Obviously, it's not something people want to endure. People who have an allergy to one form of insulin should switch to another.

Today many animal insulins have been purified, meaning they are manufactured with fewer impurities, so allergies are less common. The purest insulins are the human insulins, made through the high-tech processes we mentioned earlier. (Just for the record, today's animal insulins are 99.99 percent pure; human insulins are 99.999 percent pure!) Since the semisynthetic and synthetic human insulins are chemically identical to the body's own insulin, they do not cause allergic reactions. More and more people with diabetes are using human insulins—which, not surprisingly, are more expensive than the older beef- or pork-derived insulins.

Q: Are there other differences in insulins?

A: Yes. Insulins vary in three important ways: how quickly the insulin takes effect (doctors use the words **onset** and **absorbency** when talking about this), the intensity of effect or activity it creates (**degree**), and how long the effect lasts (**duration**). For example, human insulins have a more rapid onset and shorter duration of activity than pork insulins. Beef insulins have the slowest onset and longest duration of activity.

All three of these factors are important, but people with diabetes are often most concerned with onset and absorbency.

Q: Why is that?

A: As we noted, onset and absorbency have to do with when the insulin takes effect. A person with diabetes needs to know when the insulin kicks in, because her meals are planned around the presence of an appropriate insulin boost. Without that insulin, someone who is insulin-dependent can't absorb and convert carbohydrates and sugars into energy.

It's always a challenge to predict accurately how quickly insulin will take effect. A person with diabetes can't be sure insulin will absorb at the same rate after each injection. In fact, absorption time differs an average of 25 percent! So many factors influence how well and how quickly insulin is absorbed.

Q: Such as?

A: Foremost is the insulin itself. Absorbency differs from manufacturer to manufacturer, even within the same form of insulin. That's why insulin users generally stick to the same form (short-, intermediate- or long-acting), the same species (human, beef, pork), and the same brand (manufacturer) as long as possible.

Another important factor—and one that the individual has control over—is the injection site. Insulin is absorbed at different speeds, depending on where it is injected. Injection in the abdomen has the fastest rate of absorption, followed by arms, thighs and buttocks. Depending upon the person, the lag time for the abdomen might be 30 minutes, while in the thigh it might be 45 minutes. Exercising the arm or leg after injection increases the speed of absorption. In addition, insulin works faster when it's injected in lean areas rather than fat, which is why injection into the buttocks offers the slowest absorption rate.

Q: Which is better—fast absorption or slow?

A: That's entirely up to you and your meal plan. As long as you know the anticipated result, you can calculate when and where to inject your insulin.

Q: Sounds like a complicated proposition, keeping up with all the factors. Are there any more?

A: Yes. Injection techniques, exercise, stress, traveling, hormonal changes (such as menstruation or puberty), and even a person's metabolism affect insulin's onset, degree and duration and, as a result, his blood-sugar levels.

Q: How about the size of the dose—
does that matter?

A: Yes, as a rule, dosage varies from person to person.
Insulin comes in concentrations of 40, 100 or
500 units per milliliter (written as U-40, U-100 and U-500).
Most people use U-100. The appropriate dose depends on
the way an individual's body responds to her planned diet
and exercise regimens. Virtually all type-I and many type-II
patients need two or more injections daily to prevent blood-
sugar levels from getting too low during the day while
maintaining blood-sugar levels through the night.

Q: Now you're going to tell me that, along with
everything else she has to contend with, a
person with diabetes must plan around specific
times of the day for her injections, right?

A: Right. Once again, the best time for an injection
depends on blood-sugar levels, food consumption,
exercise and forms of insulin used.
Generally, doctors recommend an interval of 30 minutes
between injection of short-acting insulin and a meal. They
discourage people from eating within a few minutes after (or
before) injecting short-acting insulin, because that substan-
tially reduces the insulin's ability to prevent a rapid rise in
blood sugar and, thus, increases the risk of hypoglycemia a
few hours later. The consumer and her health-care practitioner
can set up guidelines for the suggested interval between
insulin injection and mealtime based on factors such as
blood-sugar levels, site of injection and anticipated activity
during the interval.

Q: Whew! This is a lot of information to have to
juggle at one time. Is there anything that can
help make this juggling act easier?

A: Yes. Your physician should set up a daily treatment
plan, which spells out elements like dosage, insulin
concentration, type of syringe and timing of injections.

He should also prepare an **algorithm** for a diabetic patient—a simple mathematical chart that can serve as a guide for determining how many units of insulin to take and when to take them, depending upon blood-sugar level. There's one hitch to using an algorithm, however.

Q: And what's that?

A: The person must regularly test her blood-glucose levels.

Q: What kind of test?

A: This regular testing is called self-monitoring of blood glucose, or SMBG. We mentioned it briefly in Chapter 1, and we discuss it in depth in Chapter 5. Basically, it's a way of monitoring blood-sugar fluctuations throughout the day, so that the person with diabetes can do a better job of reaching target blood-sugar levels.

Q: How would I do self-monitoring?

A: In a nutshell, you use a blood-glucose meter (available at most corner drugstores) to measure the blood-sugar level in a drop of your blood. The test takes 45 seconds to two minutes to give results. With the blood-glucose measurement literally in hand, you then look at your algorithm for guidance on how many units of insulin to inject.

The algorithm is a handy tool. If you don't have one, ask your doctor to create one. Because each algorithm varies from person to person, you can't follow anyone else's. An algorithm also needs constant reevaluation and occasional updating, since diabetes is one disease that doesn't stay still.

From time to time, you and your doctor may find that a change in species or brand of insulin may be necessary to keep pace with the current path of your disease.

Q: **What about that insulin? Are there certain things that I should be looking for when purchasing insulin?**

A: The most important step is to double-check the bottles to be sure you are getting the correct type, strength and brand. This is particularly important if you purchase premixed insulins, because they can be prepared in all sorts of combinations.

Pharmacists are not supposed to change your insulin preparations in any way without your doctor's approval—or without informing you—but mix-ups can happen. When you go shopping for insulin, take along an empty bottle. Or keep a copy of a label in your wallet to help you verify that you have the right stuff.

Finally, check the expiration date before you leave the store. Will you be able to use all the insulin before it expires? If not, ask for another bottle with a different shelf date.

Q: **How often must I use insulin?**

A: The answer depends upon what blood-sugar levels you and your doctor are trying to maintain.

Basically, there are two types of diabetes therapy. The first is known as the **standard**, or **conventional**, **therapy**. It's been used for decades.

The second, newer therapy is called **tight control** or **intensive therapy.** As the names imply, this therapy strives for tighter control of blood-sugar levels, and generally that means striving for less fluctuation in sugar levels.

Q: Which therapy is better?

A: We wish there was a definite answer, but you've put your finger on one of the most hotly debated aspects of diabetes care today. Physicians hold a confusing range of positions for and against tight control. Many doctors even disagree on what the term "tight control" means. We'll see why in a moment.

To settle at least part of the debate, a group of doctors and scientists are conducting a large research trial to investigate the merits of tight control. Known as the Diabetes Control and Complications Trial, this project gives a definition of tight control, which we use in this book. Basically, they define a tight-control regimen as one in which people with diabetes strive to maintain near-normal blood-sugar levels by either going on an **insulin pump** (we'll talk about this shortly) or by taking four to six insulin injections daily and performing at least four self-administered tests of blood-glucose levels per day.

Q: How different is that regimen from standard treatment?

A: Standard diabetes treatment generally entails two insulin shots a day. The **mixed-split regimen** (mixtures of intermediate-acting and short-acting insulin given before breakfast and dinner) is the most commonly used conventional regimen. Along with this comes self-monitoring of blood glucose one or two times a day.

The advantage of standard treatment is that it's a fairly easy regimen to follow. The drawback is that it's fairly inflexible. Once you take your morning insulin, for instance, you can't change the time of your meals or their size—at least not without throwing blood-sugar levels out of whack. It's difficult to make spur-of-the-moment changes and still keep blood sugar under control.

Q: So is that why an intensive therapy of tight control was developed—to remedy some of the drawbacks of standard treatment?

A: Generally speaking, yes. One of the goals of tight control is to make the diabetes treatment program more responsive to a person's lifestyle, rather than changing a lifestyle to fit his treatment program. With the technique of tight control, a person with diabetes takes more frequent, smaller injections of insulin each day. As a result, he has a great deal more flexibility in the timing of meals and exercise. Many doctors believe that when a patient has more flexibility, he is more likely to follow a treatment approach.

A second goal of the intensive, tight-control therapy is to achieve better control over blood-sugar levels, enabling a person to maintain more stable and even lower sugar levels. And it works, if he is willing to invest a lot of time and energy in a demanding routine of frequent injections and blood tests day after day after day. But many people physically feel better with a tight-control regimen, and they like the sense of empowerment they gain from being able to keep their blood sugar in a narrow range. For them, the feeling and sense of power are worth the extra effort.

Q: But you said that tight control is controversial. Why is that if the regimen helps people feel better?

A: For one thing, many people with diabetes don't want to devote that much effort to managing their disease. They are used to the standard regimen of two shots a day, and they don't want to spend more time testing their blood-sugar levels and injecting insulin more frequently.

But the big concern and the source of much of the controversy with tight control is that blood-sugar levels can get too low, leading to hypoglycemia. Also known as an insulin reaction or a low-blood-glucose attack, hypoglycemia is caused by too much insulin in the bloodstream. As we mentioned in Chapter 1, early symptoms of hypoglycemia include trembling, hunger, weakness and irritability. If blood glucose drops too low, a person may pass out, go into a coma and eventually die.

Q: What factors can cause low blood sugar?

A: Several things can provoke hypoglycemia:

- Delaying or skipping a meal
- Not eating enough carbohydrates in a meal
- Suddenly increasing exercise
- Taking too much insulin

We talk more about hypoglycemia and how to treat it in Chapter 4. But for now, it's enough to say that it's a situation people need to avoid.

Q: Are you saying that people on tight control are more likely to get hypoglycemia?

A: No, *we're* not saying it—the experts are. As early as 1990, the Diabetes Control and Complications Trial reported that people following an intensive therapy of tight control were three times more likely to experience severe hypoglycemia—in other words, reactions so intense that they required the assistance of another person to recover.

Q: If this can happen, then why do doctors support tight control?

A: Many well-known physicians (including Gordon Weir, M.D., medical director of the Joslin Diabetes Center in Boston) stand squarely behind tight control, despite the likelihood of hypoglycemia. Proponents argue that patients on tight control can achieve admirably low and stable blood-sugar levels.

Proponents of tight control also point out that the research has not demonstrated that frequent bouts of hypoglycemia pose long-term hazards. And they see tight control as the better approach until science comes up with a better treatment for diabetes.

Q: So what's the argument against tight control?

A: Opponents of tight control claim that it is "patient and physician labor-intensive, expensive to implement and potentially dangerous with no proved benefit," in the words of David Nathan, M.D., a principal investigator with the Diabetes Control and Complications Trial. Speaking in *Medical World News*, Dr. Nathan advised that physicians should be cautious about using intensive therapies until the results of the trial come out in the mid-1990s. His greatest concern is that physicians who are not experienced in managing intensive therapy may encounter an even greater risk-to-benefit ratio than that documented by the trial so far.

For those reasons, many physicians are taking a wait-and-see approach. If some of their patients request intensive therapy, they may cautiously tighten control. But for the time being they continue to advocate average control until more data are released.

Q: Let's say I start a tight-control regimen, with frequent doses of insulin. Do I have to worry about drug interactions?

A: As a smart consumer, you should discuss potential interactions anytime you take more than one medication, be it a prescription drug or an over-the-counter preparation. Public Citizen's *Health Letter* warns that even aspirin, cold remedies, antacids, laxatives and smoking deterrents (such as nicotine patches) may affect the way insulin works, so that your dose of insulin may have to be adjusted. When in doubt about interactions, ask. When not in doubt, double-check!

Q: Okay. Here's another scenario. What if I'm sick? Do I stop taking insulin?

A: The answer is a most emphatic *no*. Illness changes the effect of insulin. In some cases, you may be able to reduce your insulin dose, but most of the time you'll need to take more insulin. Call your doctor for instructions on adjusting your treatment. Blood sugar can skyrocket during an illness, especially if you have a cold, flu, infection or injury.

Q: Some people have told me to refrigerate my insulin; other people tell me not to. What's best?

A: Most practitioners recommend that you keep your insulin bottle at room temperature, because cold insulin can be painful when injected and may not be absorbed as well. Insulin remains stable—in other words, usable and effective—up to three months without refrigeration.

A few practitioners, however, recommend that you refrigerate the bottle you're currently using. Their advice is based on evidence that unrefrigerated insulin sometimes loses potency after the bottle has been in use for more than 30 days. The loss in potency is slight, which is why most doctors don't believe that refrigeration is necessary.

All the experts do agree on two things: People with diabetes should have on hand a spare bottle of each type of insulin used, and vials of insulin not in use should be refrigerated. But don't freeze them, and be sure to keep them away from heat and direct sunlight.

Q: How can I tell if insulin has lost its potency?

A: There are a few obvious indicators:

• The expiration date has passed. If so, open a new bottle.

• The bottle has been open and unrefrigerated for more than three months. If you store insulin at room temperature, write the date on the bottle when you open it.

• The insulin looks different. Inspect insulin before you use it. Has it changed in color or clarity? (In general, short-acting insulin is clear and other insulins are uniformly cloudy.) Is there a sediment on the bottom of the bottle? Have small lumps or clumps formed? A yes answer to any one question signals a loss in potency.

Q: Okay, I've checked my insulin and it looks fine. How do I load the syringe?

A: Talk with your health-care provider about the fine points of technique; injection methods are best demonstrated one-on-one. In addition, reread the instruction sheet that you should have received when you purchased your insulin and syringes. But to answer your question, we'll review a few basics:

Clean your hands and the injection site before each injection. Wipe the top of the insulin vial with 70 percent isopropyl alcohol. For all insulin preparations except short-acting, the vial should be gently rolled in the palms of the hands (not shaken) to resuspend the insulin. Don't shake it—that might cause loss of potency. After the insulin is drawn into a syringe, check the insulin for air bubbles. Give the upright syringe one or two quick flicks with the forefinger to encourage air bubbles to escape. Bubbles decrease the size of the dose.

Ask for help if you're not feeling confident about using a syringe, because improper cleansing or injection technique may lead to an infection.

Q: Can I reuse syringes?

A: If you have glass syringes, you must sterilize them first. If you're asking about reusing disposable syringes—well, that's another issue debated in the medical world.

Disposable syringes and needles are made for one use. Manufacturers won't guarantee the sterility of reused syringes. But since the cost of disposable syringes and needles really adds up over the course of a year, many people prefer to reuse a syringe until its needle becomes dull.

Q: Is that a safe thing to do?

A: On the one hand, United States Pharmacopeia medical panels do not recommend reusing syringes and needles, according to an article in *Health Letter.* On the other hand, the American Diabetes Association acknowledges that syringe reuse appears both safe and practical for many people with diabetes. The reason, they say, is that most insulin preparations contain additives that inhibit the growth of bacteria commonly found on the skin.

Q: **Are there any reasons that I should not reuse a disposable syringe?**

A: The association says you should not reuse a syringe under any of the following conditions:
- Someone else used it.
- The needle is dull or bent.
- The needle came into contact with any surface other than your skin.
- You forgot to recap the needle.
- You have an infection or open wounds on your hands.
- The skin around the injection site is red or infected.
- You are ill or your resistance to infection is low.

Q: **You read a lot nowadays about the risk of AIDS associated with sharing needles. Is that a problem I should worry about?**

A: AIDS is not going to pose a problem if you are the only person who uses the syringe. To repeat what we've said above: You should *not* reuse a syringe if someone else has used it. Never share one! To do so is foolhardy at best.

If you plan on reusing syringes, you should have excellent personal hygiene, good eyesight and the hand-eye coordination necessary to recap the needle without accidentally sticking yourself. Otherwise, you put yourself at risk of infection. Make it a habit to periodically inspect the skin around the injection site. If you see unusual redness or signs of infection, discard the syringe and consult your doctor to see if you have an infection.

Q: If I'm supposed to wipe the top of the insulin vial with 70 percent isopropyl alcohol, should I also clean the needle with alcohol?

A: Some doctors recommend that you wipe the needle with alcohol after each use. Others argue that using alcohol to cleanse the needle offers no clear benefit, adding that alcohol may remove the needle's silicon coating and, thus, make injection more painful.

Q: Personally, I hate needles. Are there alternatives to syringes?

A: Many diabetic people accept syringes as part of their self-care, while others have difficulty overcoming their distaste of needles. The good news is that a host of alternative devices for delivering insulin are available or in development. Let's look at some of them.

INSULIN PUMPS

Q: What is an insulin pump?

A: Insulin infusion pumps, as they are more precisely called, are small, battery-operated devices that pump insulin into the body at specified intervals. They include a small mechanical motor; a display window for reading measurements; a battery; a small supply of insulin (enough for several days); and a small tube, or **catheter**, connected to a needle through which the insulin flows under the skin. Insulin pumps often have a little numerical keyboard, making some models look like modular telephones, for controlling the amount of insulin that gets dispensed.

Worn on a belt or strapped to the body, pumps release insulin at frequent, prescheduled times. Today's pumps are programmable, meaning that the pump wearer can program his pump to deliver less insulin during the period when blood sugar is likely to be down (usually the middle of the night) and more insulin for those times that blood sugar tends to rise (usually early in the morning—what is called the **dawn phenomenon**).

In medical lingo, therapy with an infusion pump is called **continuous subcutaneous insulin infusion (CSII)**. Although pumps have recently made their way to neighborhood doctors' offices, some experts insist that the therapy is still too new and that consumers should undergo it only at medical facilities with a skilled professional team (including a physician experienced in CSII therapy) capable of providing continuous care in case problems develop.

Q: Aside from avoiding syringes, what are the advantages of using an infusion pump?

A: In some patients, pumps and CSII provide the same kind of improvement in blood-sugar control as multiple insulin injections (the "tight control" we spoke about earlier). And insulin pumps, like frequent injections, provide more flexibility in mealtimes. The user can also program in an extra burst of insulin if needed.

Q: Can anyone use an infusion pump?

A: Some doctors recommend CSII only when three or four daily injections fail to control blood sugar. But other doctors see it as a matter of consumer choice.

The best candidates are people who are strongly motivated to improve their sugar levels, and who have the discipline to regularly monitor their blood-sugar levels through self-testing.

Q: There must be a downside to pump therapy. Is there any bad news?

A: Like any therapy based on a mechanical device, pump therapy can pose a few potential complications, and anyone who uses an infusion pump needs to be aware of them. For instance, undetected interruptions in insulin delivery may result in episodes of extremely high blood sugar, which is why frequent blood-sugar tests are essential. Infections or inflammation at the needle site are other potential complications; they can be minimized by careful hygiene and by changing the needle site frequently.

And then there's the issue of appearance, which is more important to some people than others. Although infusion pumps come in many sizes, most of them are about the size of a paging beeper.

Q: Will pumps be getting smaller and more inconspicuous?

A: Manufacturers are making them smaller every year. But for the most inconspicuous pump of all, the award goes to the newest development in pump therapy: the **implantable pump**, also known as the **closed-loop pump**. These small devices, which are inserted under the skin, are still in clinical trial and are not yet available to the average medical consumer.

Q: How is an implantable pump supposed to work?

A: The implanted pump is a complete unit inserted within in the body, often around the abdomen. There are no long tubes or view windows, because these little computerized pumps decide how much insulin is needed and then automatically release it. In theory, they closely imitate the insulin actions of the pancreas.

The idea is that implantable insulin-delivery pumps provide even more precise insulin delivery because they are not affected by skin temperature, exercise and other variables that affect absorption of insulin injected by syringe.

As a way of helping diabetic people achieve and maintain normal blood-sugar levels, implantable pumps seem to be developing a good track record. Research on one model found that up to 50 percent of people with type-I diabetes brought their blood-sugar levels to normal—pretty good results for insulin-dependent diabetes, according to one of the researchers. And another clinical trial of a programmable implantable medication system (PIMS) reported no surgical or skin complications, severe episodes of low blood sugar, or instances of extremely high (over 1,000 mg/dl) blood sugar.

Q: **I recall hearing about problems with implants. Have they been resolved?**

A: According to an article in the *New England Journal of Medicine*, implanted pumps had plenty of problems in clinical trials during the early 1980s. Insulin tended to collect within the pump or catheter, batteries had a short life, and mechanical failures were frequent.

Most of those problems seem to have disappeared in the implanted pumps of the 1990s. Catheter blockages are still the most common complication, but they can be overcome by changing the catheter under local anesthetic.

Q: **These sound very promising. Are there any other drawbacks?**

A: As good as they sound, implanted pumps have a rather short life span—15 to 30 months, according to several pilot studies. For the time being, at least, they are not a means of lifelong insulin delivery.

JET INJECTORS

Q: **How do these devices work?**

A: As the name implies, jet injectors use pressure to shoot insulin into the skin with jetlike speed. A bit larger than a syringe, jet injectors have no needles. Thus, they are particularly useful devices for adults who are so frightened by needles that they don't take insulin as often as directed.

Jet injection is not exactly new: It was first proposed for use with insulin in the 1950s. Today's injectors appear to be mechanically reliable and accurate. Compared with syringe injection, insulin absorption and distribution differ when administered by jet injection. In general, jet-injected insulin creates a greater decrease in blood sugar than an equal amount of insulin administered by syringe—meaning that less insulin is needed to do the job.

Q: Do these have any drawbacks?

A: Some people complain that jet injectors are cumbersome to sterilize, while others point out that jet injection is not necessarily less painful than a needle. A few doctors still have concerns about the consistency of the delivered insulin dose, but on the whole, jet injectors have an established place among the ranks of insulin-delivery devices.

INSULIN PENS

Q: How do insulin pens work?

A: Like syringes, insulin pens use needles to inject insulin. But instead of having to handle vials of insulin, the user simply pops in a cartridge of insulin, indicates the appropriate number of units of insulin, and shoots the insulin in.

As the name suggests, these devices are shaped like pens. Disposable needles attach at one end. Insulin pens are popular with people who take multiple daily injections of insulin, as in the intensive, or tight-control, regimen.

Q: We've looked at a lot of different options to syringes and needles. What about costs?

A: None of the high-tech devices we've been talking about here are inexpensive. But if they are what you need to take control—and if they help you follow your treatment regimen—then you may decide they are worth the price.

Jet injectors and insulin pens are less expensive than infusion pumps, for obvious reasons. Even so, depending upon how many syringes you use in a year, experts estimate that it may take two to five years to recoup the cost of something like a jet injector.

Insurance coverage of these devices varies from company to company, although more plans are beginning to cover the new devices when prescribed by a physician.

Q: What's down the road?

A: Researchers are talking about developing an insulin pill, and one pharmacologist at Texas A & M College of Medicine predicts that the day is coming when people may take insulin through an eyedropper. But both these concepts are still under study, and results won't be seen for many years.

Until then, people with type-I diabetes need to maintain a careful balance of insulin and diet. In the best interests of their health, they need to keep an eye on new treatment methods and be aware of the complications that type-I diabetes often causes. But the most important step is to work to maintain normal blood-sugar levels. There are lots of ways to do this, as the rest of this book demonstrates.

3 TYPE-II DIABETES

Q: Which is the more serious condition, type-I diabetes or type-II diabetes?

A: The one thing both forms of diabetes have in common is high blood sugar, and that's serious regardless of the kind of package it comes in.

However, type-I diabetes is considered to be more severe, primarily because it arises swiftly and can be life threatening. As you may recall from our discussion in Chapter 1, type-I diabetes is caused when the pancreas does not produce insulin. Since the body needs insulin to turn food into energy, people with type I diabetes absolutely must take insulin in order to live. That's why they are called insulin dependent. Without insulin, these people are also at risk of ketoacidosis, a deadly buildup of poisons in the bloodstream that can develop in a matter of days.

Q: So do those of us with type-II diabetes have to worry?

A: Yes. Type-II diabetes is equally hazardous. It just poses a different sort of danger, and that is to long-term health.

By now, you know that people with type-II diabetes still have the ability to produce insulin, but that insulin no longer functions properly. People with type-II diabetes are called non-insulin-dependent, even though many of them eventually rely on insulin, at least for a time, to manage their disease.

Q: So how is this dangerous?

A: Type-II diabetes accounts for 85 to 90 percent of all cases of diabetes. In the United States, that translates to somewhere around 12 million adults. Working with all these people has given the medical profession plenty of time to find out about the long-term characteristics of this disease.

And they have found that type II is more insidious—meaning that it can proceed undetected for many years. Scientists estimate that the onset of type-II diabetes can be as quick as 4 to 7 years—or as slow as 9 to 12. Because the symptoms aren't dramatic, no one notices its presence. Unfortunately, in that time the high sugar levels associated with the diabetes may have set the stage for some serious problems, particularly heart disease and circulatory problems. Someone with diabetes, for example, is twice as likely to have a history of heart attack or stroke than his nondiabetic peers. In fact, the longer someone has the disease, the greater the risk of experiencing a related illness.

Q: Do that many people with type-II diabetes really get a related illness?

A: Consider these figures: In 1986, 144,000 people died as a result of type-II diabetes, and 951,000 were totally disabled. In 1986, the economic cost of type-II diabetes in the United States was estimated at $19.8 billion. Of that, $4.8 billion was spent on treating related conditions and complications—primarily cardiovascular conditions that manifested themselves in heart attacks, hardening of the arteries and strokes. Circulatory problems, such as poor circulation in the feet, leading to amputation, are also common in type-II diabetes.

Q: Strokes, heart attacks, hardening of the arteries, amputations—these sound like the problems of the elderly, don't they?

A: That's an astute observation. Many of the complications of diabetes are the same ones associated with advanced age. People with type-II diabetes already have one strike against them, and that's the disease itself. Some people gain another strike by living an unhealthy lifestyle.

All this is evidence of what we've noted before—that diabetes hastens the wear and tear on many crucial bodily functions.

Q: Do all people with type-II diabetes experience this wear and tear?

A: To greatly varying degrees, yes. Through scrupulous attention to a healthy lifestyle and a strong commitment to maintaining target blood-sugar levels, diabetic people can significantly slow down the degenerative process. There are a lucky few who have their blood sugar in such control that it's almost as though they no longer have the disease.

Sad to say, however, there are no guarantees. Someone may be the model of self-care and discipline yet still experience a major complication; another person who has always had zigzagging sugar levels may live to a ripe old age. There's no way around it: Life isn't just. But all the experts are adamant: The time a diabetic person spends on self-care does indeed help to minimize complications down the road.

Q: Okay, okay—I get the picture. You're basically telling me that type II is just as serious as type I, right?

A: Right. Strangely enough, though, you may run across a few members of the medical profession who don't see type-II diabetes as being just as serious, let alone who convey the message to their patients.

Q: Why is that?

A: Call it a professional prejudice or old-fashioned ignorance, but it's an attitude that does many patients a great disservice. Perhaps it's a holdover from the early days of the century, before insulin was discovered in 1921, when people with type-I diabetes died young.

Today doctors know that type-II diabetes seems mild and nonthreatening in the short term, but all the while a slow and steady destruction may be taking place. Nonetheless, vestiges of the early preference for treating type-I patients still lingers in the collective memory of the American medical establishment. In some cases, it manifests itself in the undertreatment of diabetes.

Q: Undertreatment? What do you mean by that?

A: By that, we mean that both physician and patient don't give diabetes the attention it deserves. Sometimes the complications of type-II diabetes—high blood pressure or foot infections, for example—get more attention than the disease itself.

Naturally, some attention is better than none, but only just a little better. Undertreatment is not likely to halt the slow deterioration that years of elevated blood sugar cause.

Q: So, what does this mean to me?

A: All of this plays up the importance of self-care, of taking responsibility for managing your disease. And as we've hinted, this often means changing your lifestyle. That's what this book is all about—taking charge! Granted, that's not always easy to do. But when you look at the other option—unchecked diabetes and its ultimate consequences— the decision becomes easier to make.

Q: I get the message about taking diabetes seriously. But I'd really like to know more about the disease itself. What can you tell me about the mechanics of type-II diabetes?

A: The more the medical world studies type-II diabetes, the more scientists learn that it works in various ways. Scientists now think type-II diabetes has several components. Writing in the journal *Postgraduate Medicine*, Priscilla Hollander, M.D., describes these components as:

- an inability of the pancreas to produce insulin
- an abnormal production of glucose by the liver
- insulin resistance, or a problem with the way insulin functions in the body.

Q: Do all people with type-II diabetes have all these components?

A: Not necessarily. An individual may have one, two or three, but the most common component by far is insulin resistance. Virtually all people with type II have this form of metabolic malfunction.

INSULIN RESISTANCE

Q: You mentioned insulin resistance before, but I found it a confusing concept. Would you go over it again?

A: Sure thing.
    Insulin resistance is a term used to describe this situation: The pancreas makes insulin, but for some reason the insulin is not very effective at transferring glucose from the blood into the cells of the body. Sound confusing? We can give you a more vivid description of how this works.
    Imagine your cells as little orbs powered by that form of sugar known as glucose. On the surface of these orbs are tiny structures, called receptors, that serve as gateways to the cell. In order for a cell to absorb glucose, its gateways must be

open. Insulin is the hormone that opens those gates by latching onto the cell at its **receptor sites**.

Several problems can develop in people with type-II diabetes. First, the number of receptors on each cell is lower than normal. Second, some of the insulin is not able to latch onto the receptor sites—in effect, these people's cells are resistant to their body's insulin. Third, the pancreas' insulin-producing capacity declines.

There are other theories to explain the mechanics of type-II diabetes. However, in the end, the cells don't absorb enough glucose from the bloodstream, so high blood-sugar levels develop.

Q: So if I understand you correctly, you're saying that people with type-II diabetes have plenty of insulin in their bodies?

A: Very often, people with type-II diabetes have normal or even above-normal levels of insulin.

Q: Above normal? How does that happen?

A: Think of those beta cells in the pancreas, trained to respond whenever blood sugar goes above a certain level. When blood-sugar levels build up because insulin isn't doing its job well, the beta cells cheerfully pump out more insulin. But still that insulin doesn't get used efficiently.

In some people, a high level of insulin eventually builds up in the blood, a situation that doctors call **hyperinsulinemia**.

Q: Is that a problem?

A: That's something doctors wonder about. It's been suggested that insulin itself may contribute over the long term to **vascular** disease—in other words, problems with blood vessels (such as hardening of the arteries, a condition known as **atherosclerosis**). But many doctors point out that such concerns are "based on speculation with little supporting data," in the words of diabetes expert Dr. Hollander.

Q: Okay, you've explained that type-II diabetes can be caused by several problems related to insulin and blood sugar. But why do people develop these problems in the first place?

A: Scientists have linked type-II diabetes to two predisposing factors. The first is fairly obvious.

HEREDITY

Q: You mean heredity, don't you?

A: Yes. Type-II diabetes often runs in families, suggesting that some genetic trait puts people at greater risk of developing type-II diabetes.

Q: Do doctors have any idea of what that genetic trait may be?

A: Well, yes. A recent article in the *New England Journal of Medicine* hypothesizes that a defect in the way in which skeletal muscles convert glucose into **glycogen** (the form in which glucose is stored for later use) may underlie the development of type-II diabetes. The medical literature is full of many other similar theories that strive to unravel the minute mysteries of type-II diabetes. But a discussion of those theories is a tad too technical for our purposes.

Instead, we need to focus on one key point: You are not born with insulin resistance or type-II diabetes—but you may be born with the ability to develop type-II diabetes. And this leads us straight to the next influencing factor.

OBESITY

Q: Which is . . . ?

A: Being overweight. Intimately related to this is overeating, which in and of itself can exacerbate type-II diabetes.

In fact, obesity is considered to be the primary trigger for insulin resistance and type-II diabetes. Approximately 85 percent of people with type-II diabetes are obese (20 percent or more over the ideal body weight) and, in almost all cases, the obesity preceded the development of overt diabetes.

Q: Do all overweight people eventually develop diabetes?

A: No, although many of them become insulin resistant, even though they don't develop the skyrocketing sugar levels of diabetes.

But look at it this way: Being overweight places heavy demands on the body for more insulin and contributes to insulin resistance. A person who might need about 50 units of insulin a day at a normal weight might require as much as 120 units daily to maintain normal blood sugar when overweight. The extra insulin is needed to make up for insulin resistance.

Again, some researchers argue that insulin resistance is an acquired condition, not a condition that people are born with. June Biermann and Barbara Toohey, writing in *The Diabetic's Book* (Los Angeles: Jeremy P. Tarcher, 1990), carry the point further, arguing that obesity is the disease and diabetes the complication. Whether or not you agree with that view, researchers have found that both insulin resistance and type-II diabetes can be largely reversed by successful weight loss.

Q: Do you mean that diabetes can be treated through diet?

A: Yes. Diet has been called the cornerstone of treatment for type-II diabetes. It's generally the first treatment a diabetic person tries.

DIET

Q: What kind of diet?

A: *Diet* is a bit of a tricky word. On the one hand, it means careful attention to the foods you eat. On the other hand, the word conjures up images of short-term, intensive periods of calorie deprivation that may or may not be nutritionally sound.

What most diabetes experts mean by diet is a carefully crafted eating plan—a plan that someone with diabetes can comfortably continue for life. This eating plan might be developed with the assistance of a dietitian or nutritionist. It will address not only how much food can be eaten but also the type of food eaten. Following an eating plan to improve blood sugar is known as **diet therapy**.

Q: What does it entail?

A: Diet therapy includes two strategies: calorie control and weight loss. For most people with diabetes, accomplishing both requires a complete change in eating habits—a new way of thinking about food, in effect. We discuss the ins and outs of nutrition for diabetic people in Chapter 5.

Q: What can a new eating plan achieve?

A: For someone with type-II diabetes who is not over-weight, simply controlling calories may be all that's needed to improve blood-sugar levels markedly.

In someone who is overweight, the weight loss achieved with a low-calorie diet can produce a major improvement in blood-sugar levels.

If you think about it for a minute, you can see how that works: The moment someone stops overeating, the need for insulin decreases and insulin production slows. (Remember, insulin production is stimulated each time food is eaten.)

Cutting back on food intake can immediately reduce blood-glucose levels. At the same time, the symptoms of diabetes—intense hunger and thirst, fatigue, frequent urination—begin to disappear within a few days, and even before the person has lost an ounce of weight!

Q: Why does this happen so quickly?

A: It's theorized that proper diet helps insulin receptors work more effectively. In a sense, they're not constantly being overwhelmed by calories.

Q: You've been talking about using diet to lower blood-glucose levels. Just what kind of blood-glucose numbers should people with diabetes aim for?

A: Many years ago doctors set very modest treatment goals. At that time, the major thrust was to treat the symptoms of diabetes—particularly polyuria (frequent urination) and excessive thirst—and to lower fasting-blood-sugar levels to under 200 mg/dl.

Doctors have since learned more about the long-term complications of type-II diabetes. Today they encourage their patients to strive for a more ambitious achievement—the same target blood-sugar levels aimed for by people with type-I diabetes.

Q: And what are those targets?

A: Targets vary from person to person. Some doctors set a narrower or slightly different range than we're showing here, according to their philosophy of practice. But as a rule of thumb, targets include blood glucose in the range of 70 to 120 mg/dl in the morning before eating; 180 to 200 mg/dl one hour after a meal; and 70 to 130 mg/dl three hours after a meal. Obviously, these are much lower blood-glucose levels than were aimed at years ago.

Again, targets should vary. Each diabetic person and his physician must set a realistic goal.

Q: How much weight does someone need to lose to see blood-sugar improvements?

A: Not as much as you might think. A 10 percent weight loss is the figure we've most often come across. Depending upon the individual's weight, that may mean as little as 10 pounds. As one physician puts it, the goal of weight loss is to decrease insulin resistance, and a person with diabetes doesn't always have to reach his ideal weight to improve blood-sugar levels.

The point is, any amount of weight loss is good, because it immediately decreases the amount of insulin you need.

Q: Besides losing weight and consuming fewer calories, are there other things a person with type-II diabetes has to do related to diet?

A: Actually, yes. Many people with type-II diabetes also have **hypertension** (high blood pressure) and **hyperlipidemia** (a high level of fat in the blood). Both hypertension and hyperlipidemia are associated with an increased risk of heart disease—just what you don't need. In addition, high blood pressure strains the heart, wears down the arteries and increases the risk of stroke, heart attack and kidney problems.

Hypertension and hyperlipidemia are both affected by the type of foods people eat. In Chapter 5, we discuss the foods that should be avoided to keep blood pressure and blood fats down.

Q: How many people control diabetes strictly with diet?

A: Not enough, unfortunately. Statistics published in *Postgraduate Medicine* paint a rather sobering picture: At the end of one year, only 10 to 20 percent of people with type-II diabetes are able to bring their blood-glucose levels down to normal through diet. Within five years of diagnosis of their disease, around 90 percent with type-II diabetes need another treatment method.

Q: Why is the success rate so low?

A: Wish we knew! Doctors often say it's primarily because their patients are unable to lose weight or to control the amount of calories ingested. It could be the success rate would be much higher if more people with diabetes combined a change in eating habits with an earnest commitment to exercise. The medical books often list exercise as being the second step in the treatment of type-II diabetes, but ideally it should be part and parcel of diet therapy.

Q: Why is exercise important?

A: Exercise itself helps reduce blood-glucose levels and makes insulin more effective. Exercise also helps people lose weight faster! And it helps them maintain their lower weight.

There are other suspected benefits. Exercise seems to improve insulin's sensitivity (its ability to work), reduces the dosage requirement or the need for blood-glucose medications, and reduces the risk of cardiovascular disease.

Exercise is recommended for everyone—with or without diabetes. We talk at greater length about it in Chapter 5.

Q: Can people control their diabetes simply by getting lots of exercise? Wouldn't that make all the concern about diet unnecessary?

A: Nope. Exercise alone can't control blood-sugar levels, except in rare cases. Some folks think that as long as they are exercising vigorously and regularly, they can eat as much of anything they want. Wrong! Exercise won't control blood glucose, although it does influence it. As we said before, a sound meal plan forms the cornerstone of all treatment for type-II diabetes. Everything else must build on that sound base.

ORAL THERAPY

Q: What if exercise and diet don't reduce my blood sugar? What's next?

A: If meal planning, better eating habits, weight loss and regular exercise do not keep blood sugar in your target range, then most mainstream practitioners recommend using medication to lower blood glucose. Referred to as oral hypoglycemic agents, oral hypoglycemics or oral agents, these pills are also prescribed for those people who (for whatever reason) are unable or unwilling to control their weight and food intake. The use of these pills is called **oral therapy**.

Q: What do these drugs do?

A: Oral hypoglycemics lower blood-sugar levels. They seem to do it by increasing the amount of insulin the pancreas secretes and by helping the body use that insulin more effectively.

Q: What kind of oral hypoglycemic agents are available?

A: In the United States, oral agents come from one chemical family, the sulfonylureas. The first-generation sulfonylureas became available in the 1950s; the second-generation drugs were introduced in 1984.

Q: What are these first-generation drugs?

A: There are four. We'll list them by their generic names:

- **Acetohexamide:** Usual daily dose is 250-1,500 mg.
- **Chlorpropamide:** Usual daily dose is 100-750 mg.
- **Tolazamide:** Usual daily dose is 100-1,000 mg.
- **Tolbutamide:** Usual daily dose is 500-2,000 mg.

Q: What are the second-generation drugs? And why were they developed?

A: The second generation of oral hypoglycemics are **glyburide** and **glipizide**. Glyburide is given in doses of 1.25-20 mg.; glipizide is given in doses of 2.5-40 mg.

The second-generation drugs were developed in a more potent form. The argument was that because they would be given in smaller dosages, they would be safer, would cause fewer side effects and would interact less with other drugs.

Q: Do the second-generation drugs fulfill those claims?

A: That's not yet clear. The drugs just haven't been around long enough for the experts to speak with confidence.

Q: You mentioned that only one family of oral agents is used in the United States. Are other drugs available in other countries?

A: Dozens of other oral hypoglycemics are used elsewhere in the world but are not approved for use in the United States; we don't have the space to discuss all of them here.

However, one newcomer is noteworthy. Metformin, available in Canada, is now in U.S. clinical trials. Metformin is a member of the chemical family known as the biguanides. It appears to lower insulin resistance and lower blood glucose without increasing insulin production. If clinical trials prove fruitful, metformin could soon come on the market as an alternative to the sulfonylurea family of oral hypoglycemics.

Q: If I decide to use an oral hypoglycemic, how frequently would I take it?

A: Some oral agents must be taken more than once a day; others can be taken only once daily. Your doctor will set up a schedule.

Q: Can people with type-I diabetes use oral hypoglycemics?

A: No. Oral hypoglycemics work only if the body's beta cells are already producing some insulin. Because the beta cells in people with type-I diabetes have been irrevocably destroyed, these drugs can do nothing for them.

Q: Can these drugs be used for all people with type-II diabetes?

A: You bring up an important point—oral hypoglycemics work better on some people than others. They work best on people who develop diabetes after age 40, whose disease is newly discovered and who take less than 40 units of insulin a day. In prescribing oral hypoglycemics, doctors take into account the consumer's age, weight and overall health. Oral agents aren't recommended for pregnant women, because the effect on the fetus is not known.

Q: When someone takes oral hypoglycemics, does she still have to be careful about what she eats?

A: If you mean, "Does she have to control calorie intake and eat the right foods?" the answer is "Absolutely yes!" Diet can make or break the success of oral therapy. These drugs won't work if the eating plan is neglected. It's not just a matter of increasing the dosage to make up for eating too much: Beyond the recommended maximum dosage, oral hypoglycemics are not any more potent or effective.

Someone with diabetes needs to be careful that she doesn't get lulled into a false sense of security just because her blood sugar has suddenly improved thanks to the pills. No one with diabetes can safely neglect her eating plan and exercise program or skip blood-sugar monitoring. Oral hypoglycemics do not replace a healthy lifestyle!

Q: My pills come with an insert that warns about possible cardiac risks with oral hypoglycemics. Are these drugs safe?

A: The American Diabetes Association says yes. The warning stems from a scientific study set up in the 1960s that seemed to suggest a cardiac connection. Subsequent studies have not been able to justify the initial claims of increased cardiac risk, the American Diabetes Association states.

Nonetheless, in 1989 the Food and Drug Administration recommended that all prescriptions of these drugs be accompanied by an insert mentioning this problem. If you are at all concerned, discuss this issue in more detail with your doctor.

Mind you, this is not to say that oral hypoglycemic agents are miracle drugs. They do have their disadvantages.

Q: And what are these?

A: A very important one, for starters: Anyone who uses oral hypoglycemic agents is at risk for developing very low blood-glucose levels, a situation known as hypoglycemia. Symptoms of hypoglycemia include hunger, sweating, shaking, dizziness, confusion, irritability, even nausea.

Anyone who begins oral therapy must monitor blood sugar several times a day initially. Once the person has gotten accustomed to these drugs and has brought blood glucose into the target range, he may be able to schedule blood-glucose measurements once a day or once every other day.

The thing to watch for is a blood-glucose level of 60 mg/dl or below. At that point, the patient needs to take steps *immediately* to get blood-sugar levels higher. Eating certain foods or injecting glucose are two ways to do this. See Chapter 4 for complete details.

Q: Besides the possibility of low blood sugar, are there other problems with oral hypoglycemic agents?

A: Yes. Another common occurrence is allergic reaction. A rash, hives, nausea, vomiting or cramping may be a sign of an allergy. If so, the physician may prescribe a different oral hypoglycemic.

These drugs also tend to react in a strange way with alcohol. The combination of the two may create a reaction that includes an excruciating headache, a flushed face and nausea. Although harmless, this reaction can be quite startling. Again, a different oral agent may not cause that reaction.

Q: Speaking of combinations, do oral agents react with other drugs?

A: In some cases. Any drug or medication has the potential to interact with another substance. Cortisone in particular has been known to raise blood-sugar levels and make oral hypoglycemic agents less effective. When in doubt, even about nonprescription medicines, people should consult with their health-care practitioners.

Q: I've been told not to take oral hypoglycemics during illness. Why?

A: It's not that you can't take them, it's that oral therapy may not work. That's because periods of physical stress often create a dramatic jump in blood glucose.

Q: What do you mean by "physical stress"?

A: Those times when you have a fever, cold or flu; when you have a sinus infection or a urinary-tract infection; when you've been injured; or when you are undergoing surgery.

During these times, people with type-II diabetes should use insulin (usually a human insulin) instead of oral hypoglycemics. For some folks this insulin use is temporary. After the illness has passed, they may go back to oral therapy, again monitoring blood sugar frequently at the start.

Q: I've read that sometimes, out of the blue, an oral hypoglycemic stops working. Is that so? Does oral therapy fail?

A: Yes. As handy as this therapy is for type-II diabetes, about half of the people who use it eventually stop after five or six years, simply because the drugs no longer work.

Doctors talk about this problem in terms of **primary** and **secondary failure**.

Q: What is primary failure?

A: That's when the drugs don't work in the first place. This happens about 20 to 30 percent of the time—a fairly substantial number.

When the first oral agent doesn't work, a physician often prescribes another. The patient may have better luck the second time.

Q: Then what is secondary failure?

A: This is when the drug quits working after it had been used successfully for a while. The failure may be due to an infection, surgery or severe injury, in which case the patient may once again have good luck with the drug after the ailment or injury is cleared up. In other cases, blood-glucose levels become elevated "out of the blue," to use your phrase, and the physician has to increase the dose or prescribe a different agent. No one is quite sure what causes secondary failure, although doctors say it can happen when someone stops exercising or neglects her eating plan.

Secondary failure is a real problem. Each year, approximately 5 to 10 percent of patients on oral therapy experience secondary failure. The medical world hoped that the second-generation sulfonylureas would be less vulnerable to this problem, but that doesn't seem to be the case, although results are still coming in on these new drugs. All in all, according to a report in *Medical World News*, oral agents in the sulfonylurea family fail to bring blood sugar under control in 30 to 40 percent of people with type-II diabetes.

Q: So, what happens when oral hypoglycemics fail?

A: For some individuals, insulin is the next step.

INSULIN THERAPY

Q: Insulin? But I thought only people with type-I diabetes used that?

A: Not so. Insulin is used when other therapies have failed. And to be quite honest, many diabetes therapies fail, at least according to the medical profession's point of view.

Dr. Hollander explains it this way: If achieving normal blood-sugar levels is the treatment goal for type II, then the United States has a fairly dismal track record. "Only a fraction of patients do well on diet therapy alone, and the primary failure rate of treatment with an oral hypoglycemic agent may be as high as 30 percent," she writes in *Postgraduate Medicine*. "Eventually, 60 to 70 percent of patients with type-II diabetes who are being treated aggressively need insulin treatment." She suggests that a new term be coined for these patients' disease, such as "insulin-requiring diabetes mellitus" or "IRDM."

Injected insulin helps with type-II diabetes because it gives beta cells in the pancreas a rest—after all, the disease has been forcing them to work overtime. After a period of time, when blood sugar has been controlled, the patient may be able to resume the use of oral agents.

Q: Are there any drawbacks to giving insulin to patients with type-II diabetes?

A: A few. The first is hyperinsulinemia, which we mentioned before. Giving insulin to insulin-resistant type-II patients may contribute to or exacerbate hyperinsulinemia, which may be a risk factor for cardiovascular disease.

Another area of concern with insulin therapy is its effectiveness in very overweight people. Some extremely obese type-II patients require huge amounts of insulin, and even with large doses they aren't able to control their blood sugar. In addition, insulin tends to promote weight gain, a particularly undesirable effect for type-II patients, as most of them are overweight to begin with.

Q: Are these problems common?

A: Not really. Most people with type-II diabetes do well with insulin.

Q: What do I do with the insulin?

A: We recommend that you read Chapter 2 of this book, which reviews the ins and outs of insulin injection. Most people with type-II diabetes need to take two shots of insulin a day, just like their type-I peers. Many do well taking a mixture of regular (short-acting insulin) and NPH (intermediate-acting insulin) twice a day—oftimes before breakfast and dinner—which is, again, similar to the most common regimen used by people with type-I diabetes.

Anyone—type I or type II—using insulin must monitor blood-glucose levels several times a day. The data derived from these blood-glucose readings provide the physician and diabetic patient with the information needed to make adjustments in insulin doses and to watch for instances of hypoglycemia—a common problem with insulin use.

NEW THERAPIES

Q: Are doctors developing any new therapies for type-II diabetes?

A: The newest brainchild, called **combination therapy**, is now in clinical trial. It combines oral hypoglycemic pills with one shot of insulin a day, usually a small amount of NPH late in the evening.

Many specialists see great potential in combination therapy, particularly for what they term "poorly controlled patients." One of the benefits of this therapy is that less insulin might be used. Indeed, a Finnish study found that type-II patients treated with insulin and sulfonylurea required 50 percent less insulin compared with an insulin-only group.

Another drug—metformin, which we discussed earlier—is also being explored in combination therapy. The exciting thing about metformin is that it doesn't produce hyper-insulinemia, says Alan Garber, M.D., of Baylor College of Medicine, in Houston. "All other diabetes therapies produce some degree of hyperinsulinemia, which increasingly seems related" to cardiovascular disease, he notes in the pages of *Medical World News.* Considering that 77 percent of all diabetic hospitalizations, other than for hypoglycemia, involve cardiovascular complications and that 80 percent of the deaths are cardiac in nature, it's easy to see why doctors are excited about this potential therapy.

Most investigators expect diabetes therapy to increasingly involve combination therapies. However, it may be years before they are available to the average person with diabetes.

Q: Are there any surgical approaches to treating type-II diabetes?

A: Two surgical procedures can affect diabetes but they are not really treatments for diabetes: gastric stapling and vertical banding gastroplasty. Both procedures do the same thing—they make a small pouch out of part of the stomach, thereby shrinking the size of it. Theoretically, the person who has such surgery cannot eat as much food as

before. Because these procedures affect food intake, they
affect diabetes. But—to reiterate—they are not surgical
"cures" for diabetes.

Doctors are debating the role of pancreas transplants, beta-
cell transplants, and/or use of an artificial pancreas for type-II
diabetes—the same sort of surgical approaches to type-I
diabetes now in clinical investigation and which we talked
about in Chapter 2. But those aren't options for type-II
diabetes right now, although they may be in the future. The
best tools for handling the disease still remain the most
fundamental ones: diet and exercise.

Q: So it ultimately all comes back to diet, eh?

A: Absolutely. There's no reason more people cannot succeed at maintaining target blood-sugar levels
through a combination of weight loss, careful eating and
exercise. It all begins with commitment, willpower and the
realization that you, the person with diabetes, have control
over your health and your future.

Remember, one-fifth of everyone with type-II diabetes has
succeeded at controlling blood sugar through diet.

Q: Is their diabetes gone forever?

A: Not really, but as long as they maintain a healthy weight and stick with their eating plan, their blood-
glucose levels stay normal, although their blood-sugar levels
may creep up every once in a while.

For many folks, shedding pounds enables them to wave
goodbye to diabetes and to its many related conditions, such
as high blood pressure and cardiovascular disease. Diabetic
complications are the subject of our next chapter.

4 DIABETIC COMPLICATIONS

Q: Why do most people with diabetes experience complications?

A: Diabetes has widespread impact, reaching into every corner of the body and touching every system. Its effects are cumulative. The longer someone has diabetes, the greater the risk of experiencing a complication, particularly those affecting the most vulnerable areas: the eyes, the heart, the blood vessels and the feet.

There was a time in the not too distant past when diabetes was devastating. Many people with diabetes died young; others were crippled by one or another of the disease's major complications: blindness, amputation and kidney failure.

Then insulin was discovered in 1921, and people with diabetes had a tool to help keep the more debilitating complications in check. Today we know that through careful lifestyle choices, people can delay the onset of diabetic complications and slow the progression of the disease and its related ailments.

Despite these inroads, diabetic complications remain a reality for some folks. And in that lies a certain irony: Medical science now helps people with diabetes live longer, but the longer they have the disease, the greater the risk of experiencing any of a variety of related conditions.

Q: What sorts of conditions are you talking about?

A: Eye problems, for starters. Diabetes is the major cause of blindness in adults: Blindness is five times more prevalent among people with diabetes than among people with normal blood-sugar levels.

Infections and ulcers in the lower legs and feet are other diabetes-related problems. Diabetes is responsible for half of the amputations performed in the United States.

In addition, diabetes is thought to cause a quarter of kidney failures. And people with diabetes experience heart attacks or strokes twice as often as people who don't have diabetes.

How these complications develop is the subject of this chapter.

Q: How can I tell if complications are developing?

A: Generally, you can't, at least not without undergoing a test or medical procedure in a doctor's office. Diabetes proceeds unnoticed, silently ravaging the body. People with diabetes are often without symptoms until some damage is already done.

There is, however, one surefire indication that problems are developing, albeit quietly.

Q: And what's that?

A: Persistently high blood-sugar levels. In fact, you might argue (as many doctors do) that high sugar levels are the cause of the problems. It's a message that you've heard before in this book and that you'll hear again: Control of blood sugar is all-important.

Q: What is considered a dangerously high blood-sugar level?

A: Today's diabetes experts believe that, over the long haul, levels above 240 mg/dl are unacceptable. The ideal level is the target set by you and your physician. It will probably be in the 80 to 120 mg/dl range.

Q: Who is more likely to experience complications, someone with type-I diabetes or someone with type II?

A: Because people with type-I diabetes usually get the disease earlier in life than those with type II, they have the dubious distinction of running a greater risk of developing complications. For the most part, complications appear in people who have had diabetes for 15 years or more, although certain short-term complications can appear (and disappear) at any time.

Evidence of diabetes-related eye problems, for example, is present after five years in 1 percent of type-I cases; by 14 years the percentage is close to 100.

Once complications begin, they proceed at vastly different rates. The thing to remember is this: Every person is different. No one can predict where or when or even if complications will arise. You may never experience problems. But since no one can be certain, it's important to practice sound health habits.

Q: Do all people with diabetes develop these problems?

A: Individuals with type I tend to develop different problems than those with type II. For instance, type-I diabetes tends to produce vision problems sooner than type-II diabetes, while type-II diabetes appears to be linked to more heart attacks and strokes.

Q: Why these differences?

A: Scientists don't really know. Nor do they know why complications sometimes develop in people who have blood-sugar levels firmly in hand while other people never develop complications, regardless of how well or poorly they control their blood sugar. It may boil down to genetic differences or even to factors yet unknown.

Q: Will an individual with diabetes develop all these complications?

A: It's entirely possible to experience several types of problems—vision and feet problems, for example. But it's rare indeed to see all diabetic complications in one person.

Q: Is there any way to prevent these problems?

A: Experts believe that good control of diabetes, beginning from the first day diabetes is diagnosed, may prevent many of the common diabetes complications and lessen the severity of other complications. In fact, many people who begin a regimen of blood-sugar control can reverse some of the temporary damage that certain complications cause.

Q: You've mentioned eye problems, blindness, amputation, kidney disease—just how many kinds of diabetes complications are there?

A: Somewhere in the neighborhood of three dozen, if you count various small conditions and infections. It may be more helpful, however, to look at these problems as falling into two groups.

Diabetes complications are classified as short term (those that strike quickly at any time) and long term (those that develop only after someone has had diabetes for years). The medical profession often uses the term **acute** when talking of short-term, rapidly occurring complications and **chronic** when referring to long-term complications.

Let's look at some of the major players on both teams.

SHORT-TERM COMPLICATIONS

Q: Are short-term complications less serious than long-term problems?

A: Not really. Short-term complications can occur at any time and can certainly can be dangerous— sometimes fatal. But the plus side of short-term problems (if you can think of problems as being positive!) is that they generally can be prevented or reversed. The most common are hypoglycemia and diabetic ketoacidosis or coma.

Hypoglycemia

Q: Hypoglycemia—you've mentioned this complication before. It's a dangerously low level of blood sugar, right?

A: Right. Usually indicated by blood-glucose readings of 60 mg/dl or lower, hypoglycemia is one of the most common complications of diabetes. People often call this an **insulin reaction**. It begins abruptly. Once the cycle of low blood sugar gets under way, it can proceed rapidly. In a matter of hours the person may go from feeling uncomfortable to becoming irritable and incoherent. The latter are signals that the brain is no longer getting enough glucose. Eventually, if the low sugar levels continue, the person may pass out and go into a coma. Left untreated, hypoglycemia can cause death.

Doctors sometimes call hypoglycemia an **iatrogenic** condition, meaning that it can be caused by the *treatment* of the disease.

Q: How can treatment cause this condition?

A: Consider the situation of someone with untreated diabetes: Her blood sugar is always above normal, so she isn't at risk of hypoglycemia, or low blood sugar. Once someone begins to treat her diabetes—in other words, using diet, exercise, insulin or medications (known as oral agents) to maintain blood sugar at normal or near-normal levels— then she is more likely to have instances when she over- shoots the mark, so to speak, and brings her blood sugar down too far.

Q: Who gets insulin reactions?

A: Insulin reactions frequently happen to people who use insulin or oral hypoglycemic agents, and it's especially prevalent in those people with type-I diabetes who follow a regimen of tight blood-glucose control. (See the discussion of tight control in Chapter 2 for more details.) As you recall, achieving a normal blood-sugar level is a deli- cate balance between sugar and insulin. Too much insulin can upset the applecart.

To be very specific, someone might take too much insulin or too large a dose of an oral hypoglycemic agent. If the overdose is not counterbalanced, very low blood-sugar levels may develop.

There are, of course, other ways that someone taking insulin or oral agents might inadvertently cause blood-sugar levels to fall too far.

Q: Such as?

A: We've mentioned these before. They include taking too much insulin, delaying or skipping a meal, not eating enough carbohydrates in a meal, and exercising too much, unexpectedly or at the wrong time of day. Drinking a large quantity of alcohol can sometimes throw blood-sugar levels out of whack.

Q: What are the signs of hypoglycemia?

A: Early symptoms of hypoglycemia include weakness, trembling, intense hunger, cold and clammy skin, sweating, quick pulse, headache, anxiety and irritability. Later symptoms include headaches, confusion and drowsiness. In severe cases, unconsciousness or seizures may occur. Treating severe insulin reactions requires assistance from another person, as the affected person can no longer help herself.

These may sound like fairly clear-cut symptoms, and for most people they serve sufficient warning. Unfortunately, many people experience a situation called **reaction denial**.

Q: Is this when someone refuses to admit she is having an insulin reaction?

A: Yes, usually because she can no longer think clearly because blood-glucose levels in the brain are too low —sometimes 20 or 30 mg/dl. In such cases a friend or family member must cajole her into drinking something sugary, such as soda, to get sugar levels up. After the insulin reaction is over, the person often looks back and says, "Yes, you were right. I did need more sugar."

There's a similar problem that isn't exactly reaction denial. It's sometimes referred to as **hypoglycemic unawareness**.

Q: What's that?

A: It's when people *don't experience* those warning signals. Those people with type-I diabetes who follow a tight-control regimen are most likely to have this problem. One team of Australian researchers studied 50 such individuals and found that they couldn't detect the warning signs of hypoglycemia 64 percent of the time when using human insulin and 69 percent of the time when using pork-derived insulin.

Q: Why don't those people experience any warning signals?

A: We've come across two explanations. The first attributes it to the fact that when someone maintains his blood sugar at near-normal levels, a drop from, say, 85 mg/dl to 60 mg/dl is not very dramatic and therefore less noticeable than, say, a drop from 240 mg/dl to 60 mg/dl that a person with unstable diabetes might experience.

Researchers offer a more technical explanation: the absence of a hormone called **glucagon**.

Q: What is glucagon?

A: It's a naturally occurring substance found in the blood, one of several so-called counter-regulatory hormones that help keep the body's sugar and insulin levels on an even keel. (Another of these counter-regulatory hormones is **epinephrine**, otherwise known as adrenaline.) Glucagon is secreted by the pancreas, and its role is to raise blood-sugar levels when those levels get too low.

In recent years scientists have found that most people with type-I diabetes gradually lose the ability to produce glucagon in response to low blood-sugar levels. This problem seems to develop during the first five years of the disease. Without this "glucagon response" to low blood sugar, people with diabetes are at high risk of severe hypoglycemic reactions, particularly with a tight-control insulin regimen. These people often display hypoglycemic unawareness, because they no longer experience anxiety, shaking or other warning signals.

Q: If hypoglycemia can cause reaction denial and hypoglycemic unawareness, then how am I to know if I have hypoglycemia?

A: There's only one way to find out: Take a blood-glucose reading. Using a home blood-glucose-measurement kit, and following the guidelines for self-monitoring of blood glucose (SMBG), you can get the real lowdown on the state of your sugar levels. Readings from the kit's blood-glucose meter can disclose what your mood or symptoms may not. (We've mentioned SMBG in previous chapters, and we thoroughly discuss this all-important self-care technique in Chapter 5.)

Q: What should be done when blood-sugar levels go down?

A: Many doctors recommend that people with diabetes eat something with carbohydrates when sugar levels get down to 60 or 70 mg/dl. Below 60 mg/dl, they should treat the situation like a medical emergency—because it could well be. Again, the first step is to eat or drink something. Traditional recommendations include drinking a small glass of fruit juice or regular soft drink (one with sugar), or eating dried fruit, six or seven Lifesavers, two tablespoons of raisins, six jelly beans or several glucose tablets. Once the reaction is treated and the symptoms subside, the person may need to eat an additional small meal or snack to prevent blood sugar from dropping again later in the day.

Your health-care practitioner can give you additional guidelines for treating insulin reactions, including a list of foods to keep near at hand. It's a good idea for anyone prone to hypoglycemia to carry a small amount of sugary foods to be eaten in the event of an insulin reaction.

Q: Let's say the person doesn't get blood-sugar levels up soon enough. What's the next step?

A: At this point, he may be disoriented, confused or even unconscious. Since you can't give food or drink by mouth to someone who is unconscious (the person may choke to death), someone will have to inject glucagon. That person might be a family member, a co-worker or a roommate.

Q: Glucagon? Isn't that one of the hormones you talked about earlier?

A: Yes. Glucagon is a naturally occurring hormone that works to elevate blood sugar. Like the hormone insulin, glucagon is manufactured by pharmaceutical companies for use by people with diabetes and, again like insulin, it is injected with syringe and needle. A glucagon injection is the way to treat a person who is unconscious because of **insulin shock**.

Q: How can I prevent insulin reactions?

A: You can monitor your blood-sugar levels frequently and act accordingly. But it's nigh on to impossible to go through life with diabetes and not experience several insulin reactions. The key is to set up a system that can help you recognize this short-term complication and to deal with it quickly and effectively when it does happen.

Ketoacidosis

Q: What is this complication, and what causes it?

A: Ketoacidosis, commonly called a diabetic coma, primarily affects people with type-I diabetes. (There's another form of diabetic coma experienced with type-II diabetes, and we'll discuss that in a moment.) Ketoacidosis is caused by a persistently high level of blood sugar, or hyperglycemia.

Certain situations enable hyperglycemia to grab a foothold:
- too much food
- not enough exercise
- not enough insulin or medication
- physical stress, such as an infection, the flu or another illness
- psychological stress

Q: A coma is dangerous, right?

A: Absolutely. Before insulin was discovered, keto-acidosis was a leading cause of death in people with diabetes. Even today, people who do not control their diabetes can die from diabetic coma. However, most people learn to recognize and treat the early stages of this complication, thus avoiding its tragic repercussions.

Q: Does ketoacidosis occur quickly?

A: No, it usually comes on slowly, over the course of many days. The situation develops like this:

Blood sugar builds up when your cells cannot absorb glucose for use as energy. At this point, the body begins to burn fat as fuel, producing waste products known as ketones. These ketones accumulate in the blood (a situation known as **ketosis**) and eventually work their way into the urine (a situation known as **ketonuria**).

As ketones continue to build up, a tremendous amount of fluid (in the form of urine) is discharged from the body and dehydration begins. The blood eventually becomes extremely acidic. At this point, ketoacidosis has set in. If untreated, ketoacidosis affects brain function, leading to loss of consciousness and death.

It might take 12 hours, it might take 36, but ketoacidosis will arrive if the person doesn't recognize his symptoms and take steps to lower his blood glucose.

Q: What are the symptoms of ketoacidosis?

A: The symptoms may include frequent urination and great thirst, fever, vomiting or nausea, blurred vision, abdominal pain, disorientation and drowsiness. Frequent urination, in particular, causes dehydration, which increases blood acidity. Unconsciousness finally results.

Q: How can someone with diabetes tell if ketoacidosis is developing?

A: When the person notices symptoms that resemble those of ketoacidosis, the first step is to test his blood-sugar levels. If those levels are over 240 mg/dl for two consecutive tests, the next step is to test the urine for the presence of ketones. Ketones are sometimes referred to as **acetones**, and the urine test for ketones is sometimes called a urine acetone test.

If both blood-sugar and ketone levels are high, the person should give himself a dose of regular, fast-acting insulin immediately and call his physician for additional instruction. In most cases, additional insulin doses and exercise can rein in this condition before it reaches the advanced stage—when ketoacidosis must be treated in a hospital.

Q: Why is that?

A: Because ketoacidosis is accompanied by dehydration, special care is needed to replace body fluids and treat the body for shock. Health-care practitioners can monitor blood glucose and other blood chemicals much more easily in a hospital setting, giving additional doses of insulin to the patient when needed. Minerals such as potassium are often very low and must be replaced gradually. When the person's blood chemistry returns to normal, he can resume his normal self-care regimen.

Q: At what point does the patient go into a coma?

A: Actually, the moniker *diabetic coma* is misleading: You don't have to be unconscious to have ketoacidosis. But to answer your question, coma can occur as the ketoacidosis advances. Obviously, it's not a good idea to let it get to that stage. Any of the symptoms plus ketones in the urine are signals to take immediate action. You can avoid a coma and even hospitalization from this short-term complication by acting quickly when blood-sugar levels are high.

Q: You said earlier that people with type-II diabetes may experience a different form of coma. What's that?

A: It's known as the **hyperosmolar**, or **nonketotic**, **coma**. Let's look at it now.

Hyperosmolar, or Nonketotic, Coma

Q: How is this different from ketoacidosis, the so-called diabetic coma?

A: This is a form of diabetic coma generally experienced by people with type-II diabetes. We should note here that some people don't distinguish between ketoacidosis and hyperosmolar comas, because the symptoms are similar and both are caused by high sugar levels. However, the hyperosmolar coma has a different chemical basis.

Q: Would you explain that in simple terms?

A: Basically, in a hyperosmolar coma, ketones do not develop, as they do in a diabetic coma. Insulin is present in the person with type-II diabetes, and even though it cannot work properly, it prevents the body from burning fat as an alternative fuel. If fat isn't burned, then ketones aren't produced. Thus the chemical difference between ketoacidosis and the hyperosmolar coma.

The cause of both comas is the same, however.

Q: **You mean high sugar levels?**

A: Yes. In a person who is insulin resistant, her body tries to lower blood-glucose levels through the kidneys, which causes the kidneys to work overtime and also causes frequent urination. A tremendous amount of fluid may be lost, causing dehydration. Although the blood doesn't become acidic, as is the case with ketoacidosis, it becomes concentrated, which is just as dangerous. Blood concentration due to dehydration is called hyperosmolar, which means "increased concentration of blood."

Q: **You said the symptoms are similar to those of ketoacidosis?**

A: Yes: frequent urination and great thirst, nausea, abdominal pain, dry skin, disorientation and, later, labored breathing and drowsiness. Ketones aren't an issue—thus the name nonketotic coma. However, like ketoacidosis, a person need not actually be in a coma to be experiencing a hyperosmolar coma—although that person will probably be disoriented and confused.

Q: **And how do I treat this problem?**

A: Again, it's important to test your blood-glucose levels regularly. If they are unusually high for several tests in a row, an insulin injection or more diabetes medication and exercise may be called for. The *Joslin Diabetes Manual* recommends that someone get immediate medical assistance when her blood sugar remains over 400 mg/dl for 12 straight hours despite additional doses of insulin. Once dehydration sets in, she may have to be hospitalized so that liquids, sugars and other blood chemicals can be stabilized.

Q: We've looked at insulin reactions, caused by very low blood sugar, and diabetic comas, caused by very high blood sugar. How can I tell these two conditions apart?

A: That's an excellent question. In the early phases of each there are differences. In general, an insulin reaction, or low blood sugar, tends to appear abruptly. The person is sweaty, with moist, clammy skin, and is nervous and edgy. Diabetic comas develop over a period of days. Someone with an impending coma will have dry skin, have nausea and be drowsy or dazed.

The thing to remember is that each person has different responses to high and low sugar. As someone with diabetes, it's wise to know what your responses tend to be. Use self-monitoring of blood glucose to track your sugar patterns and guard against these short-term but potentially deadly complications.

LONG-TERM COMPLICATIONS

Q: How do long-term complications differ from short-term problems?

A: Long-term, chronic complications take more time in developing, and once they arrive are less likely to disappear. Many long-term complications are tied to those structures that distribute blood throughout the body: the small and large blood vessels, or arteries. Although scientists are not certain how it happens, they think that years of carrying blood with high sugar levels eventually damages or impairs blood vessels. The faulty metabolism of someone with diabetes may also create some chemical change that makes blood vessels more vulnerable to damage. Either way, many diabetic complications are vascular complications—complications pertaining to blood vessels, in other words.

Let's look now at some of the major long-term complications faced by people with diabetes.

Eye Problems

Q: What kind of eye problems does diabetes cause?

A: They include minor problems in focusing, premature development of **cataracts** and various degrees of retinal damage (otherwise known as diabetic retinopathy).

Q: How common are these problems?

A: It's very likely that someone with diabetes will experience at least one of these problems in the course of his lifetime. Most people who have had diabetes for 5 to 10 years show some signs of eye damage, although it may be slight.

Q: I've heard about cataracts. They are a clouding of the lens in the eye, right?

A: Right. Cataracts are a very common problem in older people, including folks who don't have diabetes. However, the evidence suggests that diabetes accelerates cataract development, which is one reason that people with diabetes generally develop cataracts sooner than their non-diabetic peers.

Q: What makes this happen?

A: It's all part of that intricate and still incompletely understood relationship between high blood-sugar levels and aging. One popular theory posits that when people have diabetes for an extended period of time, sugar by-products begin to build up in the lens of the eye, eventually leading to cataracts.

Q: How are cataracts treated?

A: Mild cataracts are often left as they are—but an individual with diabetes is encouraged to work at keeping blood-sugar levels within the normal range, which seems to slow the accumulation of sugar by-products and, thus, slow the progression of complications.

Once severe cataracts develop, however, many **ophthalmologists** believe that the best course of action is to remove the cataract and replace it with an artificial lens, also known as an **intraocular lens**. This surgical procedure can be done right in a doctor's office.

Although cataracts certainly impede sight, they are less troublesome than another long-term complication, diabetic retinopathy.

Q: What is retinopathy?

A: It is damage to or disease of the retina, the delicate membrane that lines the inside wall of the eye. The retina responds to light and receives the image formed by the lens.

Q: What causes diabetic retinopathy?

A: In general, changes or abnormalities in the small blood vessels of the retina—changes that take years to occur.

Q: Is retinopathy common?

A: Experts estimate that 6,000 people a year develop retinopathy. It's the most frequent cause of vision

loss in Americans 20 to 74 years old. Fortunately, early diagnosis and prompt treatment often can prevent blindness.

Q: Who gets retinopathy?

A: Almost everyone with diabetes develops this complication, but the first to feel its impact are people with
type I, who frequently develop a mild form of this condition
within five years of diagnosis of diabetes. In fact, there's a
strong correlation between the amount of time someone has
diabetes and the development of retinopathy.

Q: Correlation? What do you mean by that?

A: Quite simply, the longer you have diabetes, the
greater your chance of developing retinopathy.
Within 10 years of diabetes diagnosis, half of all people with
type-I diabetes and a quarter with type II have some damage
to their retinas. By 20 years after onset of diabetes, nearly
everyone with type-I diabetes and over 60 percent with
type II have some degree of retinopathy.

Q: How dangerous is this complication?

A: Retinopathy is not something to take lightly, if you'll
pardon the pun. Among those with type-I diabetes,
retinopathy is responsible for four-fifths of all cases of blindness; among those with type II, the number is one-third.

Of course, not all cases of retinopathy result in blindness.
The condition ranges in severity from mild to advanced.

Q: You mentioned that some people develop a mild form of retinopathy. Are you saying that there's more than one form of this disease?

A: The medical profession describes two forms of diabetic retinopathy: **background retinopathy** and **proliferative retinopathy**.

Q: What is background retinopathy?

A: This mild, early form of retinopathy is characterized by gradual narrowing or weakening of the small blood vessels in the eye. Small bulges (called **microaneurysms**) develop on the vessels. Eventually a vessel may tear or break and then bleed (known in medical parlance as a **hemorrhage**).

Most folks with diabetes develop background retinopathy, but in the lion's share of the cases the condition remains at a mild level. Vision is not affected unless blood vessels break and leak fluid into the **macula**, an area of the retina responsible for sharp, fine vision—the kind of vision you need to read this book. When fluid leaks into the macula, it swells and puts pressure on other areas of the eye. This situation is called a **macular edema**, and it leads to blurred vision.

Q: Can a macular edema be treated?

A: The swelling is sometimes treated in high-risk patients (those who appear to be at high risk for blindness) with a high-tech procedure known as **photocoagulation**. This is when a precise laser beam is used to sear shut the leaking blood vessels. Photocoagulation doesn't cure retinopathy, but it can delay the loss of vision by a number of years or, in some cases, stop progression.

For the most part, however, because background retinopathy is mild, surgical treatment isn't necessary.

Q: Okay, then, what about proliferative retinopathy. How does it differ from background retinopathy?

A: As its name suggests, this severe form of retinopathy develops when a network of new, fragile blood vessels proliferates in the retina at the site of previous break-ages or hemorrhages. Over time the new, fragile vessels may tear and leak blood into the **vitreous humor**, the clear, gelatinous material that fills the center of the eye. A small amount of blood won't dim vision, but the major hemor-rhages associated with proliferative retinopathy may be large enough to affect sight, in which case they are known as **vitreous hemorrhages**.

As the eye tries to repair the damage caused by hemor-rhages, scar tissue forms. The buildup of scar tissue may eventually damage the retina, resulting in partial loss of sight, or it may displace or cause the retina to become detached, resulting in total loss of vision.

Q: Is there any way to tell that either form of retinopathy is developing—before blindness sets in, that is?

A: For the most part, people can have severe eye damage without knowing it, because the damage may not affect vision and may cause no pain. Eye examinations with a tool called a monocular direct ophthalmoscope are used to detect damage to the retina.

Q: Is this an examination my family physician can do?

A: Yes she can, although several studies indicate that physicians who are not ophthalmologists detect proliferative retinopathy in only 50 percent of the people who have the condition. That's not a particularly encouraging track record—"no better than random chance," in the words of one eye expert.

Of course, there are some obvious indications to the person with diabetes that something has happened to her eye. Partial loss of vision—even if very small—is an indication of a problem. "Floaters," "cobwebs" and "cotton wool balls" are terms that people have used to describe vision problems caused by tiny hemorrhages in the eye. A sudden, painful loss of vision may indicate a major hemorrhage. Naturally, it's best to detect retinopathy before it reaches this stage.

Q: Can anything be done for retinopathy once it reaches the advanced stage?

A: Yes. Photocoagulation—the use of laser beams— can seal leaking retinal blood vessels or reattach a detached retina. In some people, this is enough to stop the progression of diabetic retinopathy.

Vitrectomy is another, more intricate surgical procedure used in people with proliferative retinopathy. In this procedure, a physician removes the vitreous to clear out the light-blocking hemorrhage, uses microsurgery to repair the retina, if necessary, and then replaces the vitreous with a saline solution.

Q: How effective are these eye surgeries?

A: An article in the journal *Annals of Internal Medicine* explains that photocoagulation and vitrectomy prevent deterioration of vision in around 60 percent of patients. For instance, laser therapy reportedly reduces the rate of vision loss by 50 percent in people with proliferative retinopathy and macular edema, conditions that often exhibit no symptoms. Vitrectomy reportedly improves visual acuity to 10/20 or better in 36 percent of treated eyes. That's the good news.

Q: You mean to say there's bad news?

A: Well, as the wise medical consumer knows, no surgery is free of potential complications. With vitrectomy, for example, the overall complication rate is about 25 percent, according to the *Annals of Internal Medicine* article.

Q: What about taking a different tack— are there any nonsurgical techniques available to treat retinopathy?

A: Medical research is looking at ways of slowing or even preventing the progression of retinopathy.

One small Norwegian study found that people with type-I diabetes who maintained near-normal levels of blood sugar over a long period of time—at least seven years—were significantly less likely to develop severe retinopathy. The patients in this study followed a tight-control regimen, using either continuous subcutaneous infusion pumps or multiple insulin injections. (See the discussion of tight control in Chapter 2 for a refresher in what this therapy entails.)

The American medical profession is awaiting the results of the large-scale Diabetes Control and Complications Trial to refute or justify the claim that tight blood-sugar control can prevent retinopathy. The results are due in 1994 or 1995.

Q: Is there anything else that might prevent eye damage?

A: Scientists are hoping to discover why high levels of blood glucose damage the body's blood vessels. One theory is that an enzyme called an **aldose reductase**, which converts glucose into a sugar alcohol called **sorbitol**, may play a role in triggering diabetes complications. For that reason, researchers are looking into a class of drugs called **aldose reductase inhibitors**, which block the actions of the enzyme. They hope these drugs can reduce the chance of developing retinopathy and other long-term complications. Clinical trials are under way.

Although these new treatments sound promising, the key action in the here and now is getting prompt medical care for retinopathy, particularly if you have macular edema or proliferative retinopathy.

Q: **Why is that?**

A: Here's just one example: Studies have found that there is a 16 percent risk for severe visual loss if proliferative retinopathy is left untreated for two years. That may sound like a small risk, but is it really one that's worth taking? You and your doctor must decide.

Q: **Are there other things that jeopardize eyesight?**

A: Definitely. Poor blood-sugar control, high blood pressure and a history of smoking increase the risk of retinopathy and increase the chances that the condition will worsen. And as we mentioned before, people with type-I diabetes are more likely to develop severe retinopathy.

Q: **I've heard that pregnant diabetic women are more likely to develop retinopathy. Is that true?**

A: A woman with type-I, type-II or gestational diabetes who has no retinopathy before pregnancy is unlikely to develop retinopathy during pregnancy.

However, the story is different for diabetic women who already have some retinal damage when they become pregnant. About 5 to 12 percent of diabetic women with mild retinopathy will see their retinopathy worsen. Diabetic women who already have moderate to severe retinopathy are at greater risk during pregnancy. In recent studies, about 47 percent of pregnant diabetic women had an increase in severity in retinal damage, and 5 percent developed proliferative retinopathy.

Q: What causes these rapid changes?

A: They may be due to the increased levels of hormones that accompany pregnancy. Pregnancy-induced or chronic high blood pressure is thought to play a role, too. In one study, 55 percent of pregnant diabetic women who had high blood pressure in addition to retinopathy saw their retinopathy worsen, compared with 25 percent of the women who had normal blood pressure.

Q: Let's say a pregnant woman already has some sign of retinal damage. Would lowering blood-pressure levels slow the progression of retinopathy?

A: Probably, say the experts. Doctors have also found that treating a woman's retinopathy with photo-coagulation can help reduce the risk of progression *if* the laser treatment is done before she becomes pregnant.

Like all diabetic people with retinopathy, pregnant women should get regular eye examinations to monitor the course and development of this complication.

Nephropathy

Q: What is this?

A: Officially known as diabetic nephropathy, it's a type of kidney disease that leads to kidney failure. Nephropathy tends to develop in people who have had diabetes for 20 years or more. It used to be that a third of all people with type-I diabetes developed nephropathy, but today's treatment methods and the emphasis on better blood-sugar control are shrinking that percentage. People with type-II diabetes develop nephropathy infrequently.

Q: Why is nephropathy a problem?

A: We can answer that by looking first at what the kidneys do.

The kidneys are small organs located near the waist. Inside the kidneys are small blood vessels, called **glomeruli**, that act as filters, removing wastes from the blood and discharging them through the urine. Useful products, such as **protein** and glucose, are not discharged but are sent back into the bloodstream.

Nephropathy is the condition in which small arteries in the kidneys become hardened and the glomeruli become damaged (in much the same way that the small vessels of the eye become damaged during retinopathy). The kidneys ultimately fail in their job of filtering out wastes. People with kidney failure must go on **dialysis** (the use of a machine to filter blood) or have a kidney transplant; otherwise, lethal levels of wastes and toxins build up in their bodies.

Q: What causes nephropathy?

A: High blood-sugar levels, for starters. Also, high blood pressure increases the likelihood of kidney complications. Frequent urinary-tract infections add to the problem, because an infection can easily spread to the kidneys and damage them.

Q: How does someone with diabetes find out if kidney damage is developing?

A: Early warning signs include problems emptying the bladder, blood in the urine and urinary-tract infections. The disease can be confirmed through simple urine and

blood tests. Just as the kidneys lose their ability to discharge wastes, they also lose their ability to retain protein and glucose. Sugar and protein begin to show up in the urine tests in larger and larger amounts. Blood tests detect high levels of urea nitrogen and creatinine, which also indicate kidney damage.

Q: Is there any way to treat kidney problems before kidney failure occurs?

A: The wisest step for all people with diabetes is to take urinary-tract infections seriously. Talk with a doctor about what to do when they develop. Remember, infections can back up the urinary system and spread to the kidneys, impairing their function.

If signs of developing kidney problems are detected, doctors often emphasize a regimen of tight blood-sugar control and a low-protein diet (see Chapter 5) to ease some of the stress on the kidneys.

If nephropathy progresses, however, the affected person may ultimately have to undergo kidney dialysis. Kidney transplantation is another option for some.

Cardiovascular Complications

Q: What do you mean by "cardiovascular complications"—and how are they related to diabetes?

A: The word **cardiovascular** means "of the heart and blood vessels." Cardiovascular complications are problems such as angina, heart attack, stroke and others related to poor circulation.

Just as diabetes changes the shape of the small blood vessels (known as **microvascular** changes), it also appears to thicken and obstruct the walls of the large blood vessels, thus restricting blood flow. These are called **macrovascular** changes. Macrovascular changes (such as hardening of the arteries) have been called the "underlying event" behind most cardiovascular disease. There's no doubt about it—cardiovascular complications are very debilitating side effects of diabetes.

Q: Who is at risk of developing heart attacks and strokes?

A: Just having diabetes increases a person's risk of experiencing a stroke, according to the *American Journal of Epidemiology*, regardless of whether or not the person has other risk factors.

Q: What other risk factors exist?

A: Neglecting exercise, eating a high-fat diet, having high blood pressure and smoking cigarettes—each of these confers more risk. High blood pressure alone is a major cause of strokes.

Q: I've read that heart attacks and strokes are more common in people with type-II diabetes than in those with type-I diabetes. Why is that?

A: Ah—yet another question that medical science can't completely answer. It could be because people with type-II diabetes tend to be overweight. (Obesity is a known risk factor for heart attacks.)

Q: Are cardiovascular complications more common in men than in women?

A: In the general population, yes: Women experience strokes and heart attacks less frequently than men. Among people with diabetes, however, the answer to that question is no. Men and women with diabetes, particularly with type-II diabetes, suffer equally poor outcomes after heart attacks. They have a much higher cardiovascular death rate than people without diabetes, and they are less likely to survive a heart attack than their nondiabetic peers.

Q: That's strange—women generally seem to have a biological advantage. Why does diabetes change that?

A: Diabetes appears to be the great equalizer of the sexes, at least where heart attacks are concerned. Compared with men without diabetes, diabetic men have about two times the average risk of developing cardiovascular disease; diabetic women have three to five times the average risk of developing cardiovascular disease.

Q: Wow—those are big differences. Besides the obvious steps of lowering blood sugar and losing weight, are there any other ways people with diabetes can help prevent heart problems?

A: Cholesterol and **triglycerides** are two other things to focus on if they wish to spare their hearts.

Q: Why is that?

A: If you've paid any attention to medical news in the past decade, then you should be aware of the role high cholesterol levels play in heart disease. A fatlike substance that comes from meat and diary products, cholesterol is found in all the body's cells and in the bloodstream. High levels of cholesterol in the blood, or **hypercholesterolemia**, have been implicated in the development of heart disease in general and **arteriosclerosis** (hardening of the arteries) in particular.

What you may not know is that people with diabetes tend to have higher blood-cholesterol levels than other people.

They also tend to have higher levels of **low-density lipoproteins (LDL)**, what some call the "bad cholesterol" because it aids in the deposit of fats on artery and cell walls. As if that wasn't bad enough, people with diabetes tend to have lower levels of the "good cholesterol," or **high-density lipoprotein (HDL)**, the substance that escorts excess cholesterol from the body. All of this is unpleasant news for the cardiovascular system.

Q: And those triglycerides you mentioned—what are they?

A: Triglycerides are another form of fat in the body. High levels of triglycerides in the blood **(hyper-triglyceridemia)** may not directly cause arteriosclerosis, but may accompany other abnormalities that speed its development.

Q: And now you're going to tell me that people with diabetes have higher levels of triglycerides, too. Am I right?

A: Right you are. Combine high triglyceride levels of 200 to 500 mg/dl with cholesterol levels between 200 and 300 mg/dl, and you have what the *American Heart Journal* calls *combined hyperlipidemia* (meaning too much fat). Triglycerides over 500 mg/dl and/or cholesterol levels over 300 mg/dl are called *massive hyperlipidemia*. Combined and massive hyperlipidemia are found in over 30 percent of all people with diabetes—and approximately two to three times more frequently than in people without diabetes.

We'll talk more about cholesterol and triglycerides in the next chapter when we examine diet. For now, it's enough to say that any person with diabetes who improves his cholesterol picture can protect against developing cardiovascular problems. Evidence suggests that for every 1 percent reduction in blood-cholesterol level, there is a 2 percent reduction in coronary-artery disease.

Q: Is there anything else people with diabetes can do to guard against heart attacks?

A: The medical world has found that some benefit by popping a simple pill—aspirin.

Q: Aspirin? Why is that?

A: A curious thing happened during the course of a clinical study known as the Early Treatment Diabetic Retinopathy Study. Designed to gauge the effects of aspirin on diabetic retinopathy, the study included 3,700 people with type-I and type-II diabetes. Half took two aspirins a day, the other half took a placebo. It turned out the aspirin had no effect, positive or negative, on retinopathy. But something positive did take place: People taking aspirin were 17 percent less likely to have had a heart attack during the five years of the study.

Aspirin can't solve all the cardiovascular woes of someone with diabetes, nor is aspirin use for everyone. But it would be worth a trip to the doctor to discuss what aspirin can do for you.

Neuropathy

Q: What is this?

A: Quite simply, neuropathy is nerve damage. The word *damage* suggests something irrevocable and perma-nent; actually, this is one long-term complication of diabetes that can appear and disappear in a short period of time. It also varies in intensity, ranging from mild discomfort to severe, disabling pain.

Q: What causes neuropathy?

A: As is true about many diabetes complications, the answer to this question has the medical profession stumped. It's thought that something interferes with the body's nerve pathways so that nerve impulses are no longer transmitted properly. The culprit may be uncontrolled blood-sugar levels (although many people with good control develop this complication), or it may be that the nerves are somehow damaged during the metabolic changes of diabetes.

Q: Is it common?

A: Yep. It's estimated that some form of nerve damage affects 60 to 70 percent of people with diabetes at some point in their lives. Some physicians claim that it's often the first noticeable sign of diabetes, particularly in type-II diabetes. Unfortunately, neuropathy mimics many other medical conditions (as you'll see in a moment), so it's often initially diagnosed as something else.

The medical profession divides neuropathy into two forms: **peripheral** and **autonomic**.

Q: What is peripheral neuropathy?

A: The most common form of nerve damage, it's sometimes called *sensory neuropathy* because it often creates odd sensations (or, in some cases, loss of sensation) in the legs, feet and hands.

Q: Could you describe those odd sensations?

A: Certainly. They include numbness, tingling, muscle weakness and sporadic shooting pains. These sensations can be mild or they can be annoying. Some people experience double vision for short periods of time; others have great difficulty walking because of pain or because they lose some control of leg movements. Neuropathy has been known to interfere with sleep or rest.

In general, peripheral neuropathy is a temporary condition —one that disappears as mysteriously as it appears. However, it can lead to injury in cases where the person with diabetes feels no sensations of pain. This often happens on the bottoms of the feet, resulting in some of the foot problems that we'll be discussing shortly.

Q: What is autonomic neuropathy?

A: A less common complication, perhaps experienced by 20 percent of people with diabetes, autonomic neuropathy is damage of the nerves that control various bodily functions, such as the digestive system, urinary tract and cardiovascular system.

Autonomic neuropathy leads to many inconvenient problems:

• When it affects the nerves around the stomach, bladder and bowels, it can cause vomiting, constipation and feelings of bloatedness.

• When it affects the nerves that control the contraction of blood vessels, a condition called **orthostatic hypotension** may develop. This is a sudden drop in blood pressure when a person gets up after reclining.

• **Impotence**, the loss of the ability to have an erection, is also related to (although not entirely caused by) neuropathic damage.

Q: Can these problems be treated?

A: Doctors often prescribe drugs to treat the symptoms of these different problems—for example, to relax muscles if the problem is constipation. Exercise helps some people; others benefit from bed rest. Because neuropathy varies tremendously from person to person, treating this annoying condition is often a matter of trial and error.

Medications to treat or prevent nerve damage do not yet exist, although researchers are conducting studies using aldose reductase inhibitors—experimental drugs we discussed earlier in relation to retinopathy.

Foot Problems

Q: How does diabetes affect the feet?

A: Cardiovascular complications damage blood vessels and diminish blood flow to the legs and feet. Add damage to the nerves of the legs and feet through neuropathy and you've just laid the groundwork for serious foot ailments.

Q: How often do these ailments show up?

A: In about half of people with diabetes for 20 years or more. The scenario then proceeds like this: When people with diabetes lose sensation in their lower legs and feet, they are less likely to notice damage to the skin and tissues—problems like cuts, bruises, blisters, bunions, corns, calluses, ingrown toenails or even athlete's foot. Such seemingly minor injuries can blossom into an infection known as a neuropathic ulcer.

Q: Wait a minute—a blister can turn into an ulcer? How can that be?

A: Let's say you have a new pair of shoes that has chafed and rubbed one foot raw. The area is red and inflamed. Once an inflammation or infection begins, its swelling compresses the blood vessels and arteries, which are already damaged or narrowed by diabetes itself. These factors diminish the flow of blood to the irritated area, meaning fresh oxygen and infection-fighting blood cells have a more difficult time getting to the problem site.

All of this sets the stage for a serious infection. Once infection sets in, it's difficult to treat. Antibiotics, which are carried in the blood, can't reach the infected area efficiently.

Q: Do foot ulcers tend to develop in a certain area?

A: Yes. About 80 percent of these problems occur on the bottom of insensate feet.

The real danger with the combination of infection and reduced blood flow is **gangrene**. If blood flow were to be completely blocked, the cells served by the obstructed blood vessels would die. Once gangrene sets it, the only way to stop its spread is by amputation of the dead tissue.

Q: Is amputation common among people with diabetes?

A: According to an article in *Archives of Internal Medicine*, "It has been estimated that the lifetime risk of a lower-extremity amputation is 5 to 15 percent among diabetic individuals, a risk 15 times that of the nondiabetic population."

Somewhere in the neighborhood of 60,000 diabetes-related amputations are performed each year, which is half of all lower-extremity amputations in the United States. As is true with all diabetic complications, certain factors increase risk: being male, being African-American and having a history of smoking. Risk increases with age, too.

Q: Is there anyway to find out if a blood vessel is about to become blocked?

A: Blockages in large vessels, such as those of the legs, can be spotted with an x-ray called an **angiogram**. **Bypass surgery** may be performed to detour blood around the blockage. In this surgery, a piece of a healthy vein is "harvested" from an area of the body (possibly the thigh) and is attached at either end of the obstruction. The new vein directs blood to cells that had been receiving an inadequate supply. It's one method of preventing gangrene.

Q: Is there any other way to prevent gangrene and amputation?

A: Amputation doesn't have to happen. With proper foot care, many if not most amputations may well be avoided.

How to care for your feet, how to monitor your blood-sugar levels, how to design and follow a sound eating plan—in short, how to prevent diabetic complications from developing in the first place: These are the topics we cover in the next chapter. Read on!

5 SELF-CARE: PUTTING YOURSELF IN CONTROL

Q: From all that I've learned from this book, diabetes is a complicated disease. Honestly now—will self-care really make a difference?

A: Absolutely. Unlike many other illnesses, *the control of diabetes rests in the hands of the patient.* Self-care is not just important, it's absolutely essential.

This chapter (and indeed, this entire book) is designed to help each diabetic person take charge of her own treatment. Keep in mind that the overall goal of any treatment is to control blood sugar—to keep it within normal limits. Achieving that entails reevaluating your lifestyle, adopting a new meal plan and a regular exercise routine, and making a commitment to self-monitoring of blood glucose. It also entails being aware of the symptoms and dangers of the potential complications of diabetes—those problems discussed in Chapter 4.

Q: That's a lot of responsibility! Where do I begin?

A: If you have type-I diabetes, you need to understand the ways in which insulin, food and exercise affect blood sugar. Insulin we discussed in depth in Chapter 2; food and exercise are addressed in this chapter.

If you have type-II diabetes, you need to understand the role of obesity, exercise and food consumption in insulin resistance. You may have to lose weight and become physically active. These latter two things are more than a matter of looking good—they're about making it easier for your body to produce and use insulin.

Q: Isn't there any easier way around all this?

A: Alas, no. The fact of the matter remains: Managing your diabetes is demanding and, at times, difficult. It's a daily, lifelong process. But the alternative—neglecting the disease—poses such demonstrated drawbacks that most folks opt for self-care.

As we mentioned at the start of this book, the real goal is to control your diabetes, instead of letting it control you. And the encouraging news is that control is literally in your hands!

SELF-MONITORING OF BLOOD GLUCOSE

Q: How is that?

A: We're referring to self-monitoring of blood glucose, or SMBG, that hands-on method of tracking blood sugar we've mentioned several times. With SMBG, you can test your blood-sugar level at home, in the office, on the road—any place and any time, as often as you wish. It gives people with diabetes a new level of flexibility—they don't have to make a trip to a doctor's office whenever they want an accurate blood-glucose reading, as was the case years ago.

Because SMBG can provide the information needed to balance food intake, exercise and insulin or medication, it has rapidly become a mainstay of diabetes-management plans. Doctors aren't always keen on consumer self-care and self-testing, but the health-care profession as a whole has embraced self-monitoring of blood glucose. It may well be the best invention since the discovery of insulin.

Q: How do people with diabetes perform SMBG?

A: Using a special needle called a **lancet**, a person pricks his finger and then places a drop of blood either on a test strip or on a specially treated sensor pad on a glucose meter (a device about the size of a hand calculator). Some test strips change color depending upon the amount of glucose in the blood, and the color is compared to a master chart. Other strips are inserted into a glucose meter. The blood-glucose meter indicates just how many milligrams of glucose are present in a deciliter of blood. The reading appears on the meter's display panel in numbers, and the whole test is done within 45 seconds to two minutes.

Q: **Self-monitoring sounds so simple. What can it achieve?**

A: Self-monitoring is valuable for anyone who is at all concerned about managing his disease. Because the process is relatively quick, it can be done many times a day, giving the person a clear picture of how his blood glucose fluctuates throughout the day. When blood sugar slides outside of target levels, the person can take action.

Q: **Should all people with diabetes self-monitor their blood-sugar levels?**

A: These days, self-monitoring is recommended for anyone who uses insulin—whether the person has type-I, type-II or gestational diabetes. Many doctors insist that adjustments in insulin doses should be based on blood-glucose measurements. One reason is that even an identical dose of insulin will be absorbed differently from day to day, depending on factors like insulin sensitivity, exercise, stress, types of food eaten and hormonal changes (puberty, the menstrual cycle, pregnancy).

Self-monitoring is also recommended when someone begins insulin therapy or changes to a new insulin species, brand or dose. (See Chapter 2 for a review of insulin terms.) During the adjustment or transition period, the person with diabetes uses SMBG to carefully track blood-glucose levels and ensure they are within target ranges.

SMBG is also recommended for those people with type-II diabetes who are using oral hypoglycemic agents, because those folks face of the danger of very low blood sugar when using those drugs.

Further, there are additional circumstances in which doctors say SMBG is mandatory.

Q: What are those circumstances?

A: SMBG is required for people who are following a tight-control regimen, whether via insulin pump or frequent insulin injections. As we discussed in Chapters 2 and 4, people following a tight-control regimen are more able to keep their blood-sugar levels on a near-normal, even keel, but they are prone to frequent bouts of hypoglycemia, or dangerously low blood sugar. Frequent self-monitoring can flag falling blood-sugar levels before they become disruptive.

Another circumstance that calls for SMBG is illness, sometimes referred to as physical stress. Illness wreaks havoc with the body's blood-sugar levels, often increasing sugar even if someone does not eat or drink. Thus, people with diabetes generally need to take more insulin when they are sick. But how much more? The results of self-monitoring can guide them and their doctors in making that decision. In fact, in any case where they are forced to step off their regular medication plans and wander into uncharted territory, SMBG is essential—a compass in the wilderness.

Q: Do other circumstances call for self-monitoring of blood glucose?

A: People who have wide swings in blood-sugar levels often turn to SMBG to find out why. You may have heard of the term **brittle diabetes**; it describes a rare condition, generally found only among people with type-I diabetes, in which blood-sugar levels fluctuate dramatically from day to day.

Q: What causes brittle diabetes?

A: Wide swings may be caused by poor management of the disease. Or they may have at their root a completely different hormonal disorder, another disease or the side effects of drugs. At any rate, self-monitoring can help someone with diabetes track sugar swings and determine how much insulin is necessary, depending upon each day's blood-sugar levels.

As we mentioned earlier, SMBG is growing in standing with the medical profession. Your doctor may proffer other reasons to practice this simple self-care technique.

Q: You mentioned that people with diabetes can monitor their sugar levels as often as they want. Is there a required minimum?

A: Frequency is determined by the patient and her doctor, although most would agree that haphazard or infrequent measurement—say, only once a week—can give little information to go on.

That said, there are some commonly recommended measurement patterns. For instance, people just beginning SMBG may be instructed to check their blood sugar four to eight times a day, including first thing in the morning, before and after each meal and last thing before bed.

People using insulin (including people with type-I and type-II diabetes) may average four checks a day: before each meal and late in the evening.

People with type-II diabetes who have their sugar under control have the greatest flexibility. Their monitoring schedule might include a morning check four to seven times a week along with the occasional before-meal or bedtime test.

Q: Am I correct in assuming that people with diabetes generally test their blood before meals?

A: Those who use insulin need these readings to determine how much insulin to take. Some folks like to take the occasional reading after a meal (known as a **post-prandial** reading), because that's the time when blood sugar shoots up. It can help to gauge how high sugar goes after food consumption.

Q: Are there other times when people with diabetes should monitor their blood sugar?

A: To be precise, there are other times when they should monitor *more frequently* than they usually do—something that we talked about earlier. These situations include illness, changes in medication, travel or any change in routine.

Q: Would something like a change in job be included?

A: Yes—basically any change in lifestyle, including a new exercise pattern, a different diet (one that may occur when visiting friends or relatives, for example), relocation, job change, marriage, retirement.

Travel through several time zones, especially by air, makes it more difficult to time medications and meals. Here, SMBG can give a person with diabetes the information he needs for dose adjustments. (Doctors can give special advice about insulin administration when traveling great distances, such as overseas. Self-monitoring will still be important, though.)

In addition, someone can voluntarily increase the frequency of monitoring whenever he wants more information about what's happening in his body.

Q: So SMBG is primarily used for adjusting insulin doses?

A: In the short term, self-monitoring tells you what action you need to take to get blood sugar within the target range set by you and your doctor. But SMBG is also used to build a larger picture—a month-by-month, year-by-year image of what doctors call **glycemic control**, or overall control of blood sugar.

SMBG enables people with diabetes to build a data base of sorts. Toward this end, many of them start a notebook or diary and record in it the results of their blood-glucose tests. (Some of the new blood-glucose meters store this information in an electronic memory.) Over time, these details disclose how their blood sugar reacts to exercise, to certain foods, to travel and to other environmental factors. With information in hand, people then discuss results with their doctors during routine office visits. Ultimately, all of these pieces of information help fine-tune the diabetes-management program.

Another benefit of getting to know what's normal for your body is being able to spot a developing problem or emergency, such as an unusually high (or unusually low) blood-glucose reading.

Q: If I measure my blood sugar four times a day, won't that get expensive?

A: It's costly, no doubt about it. People with diabetes spend somewhere in the neighborhood of $396 million each year on blood-glucose-measuring devices alone, according to 1992 statistics. And the market for these devices is growing.

Among those who use these devices, the cost of meters and supplies averages $400 a year. Part of the price depends on your choice of equipment—necessities like lancets, test strips and glucose meters. Many of today's high-tech glucose meters have sticker prices of $50, $150 and up. Some manufacturers offer meters at steep discounts, knowing that consumers must purchase test strips or other supplies specifically developed for those meters.

New versions of blood-glucose kits arrive on the market every season. The trend is toward developing new products that make self-testing simpler, more convenient and quicker. Blood-glucose meters, for example, have become smaller and less cumbersome in recent years—good news if you're inclined to tote a meter along with you on your daily travels.

In actuality, SMBG is a small part of the total cost of diabetes care—a drop of blood in the bucket, so to speak.

Add in the cost of blood tests performed in a doctor's office (we discuss those later in this chapter), and the annual tab for blood monitoring can easily exceed $1,000—an amount covered by many (but not all) health insurers. Yet if self-monitoring delays or prevents the pain, the aggravation and the cost of diabetic complications, then that money is well spent.

Q: **Are there any measurement tools besides test strips and glucose meters?**

A: A device with a new approach to measuring blood-glucose levels is now in clinical trial. It's called an infrared blood-glucose analyzer.

Q: **What does it do?**

A: The person inserts a finger into a hole in one side of this shoebox-sized device, then the device measures current blood-sugar levels by a process called "attenuated photo reflection." In short, measurements are made without drawing blood. In one small trial, scientists found that the analyzer's error rate was about the same as the error range of standard fingerprick tests. This high-tech blood-glucose analyzer may be on the market in the mid-1990s—toting with it a price tag in the neighborhood of $2,000.

Q: **Hold on a moment—you mentioned the words "error rate" and "error range." Are you suggesting that glucose meters aren't accurate?**

A: To quote members of the medical world, a "20 percent deviation from baseline" is acceptable. Translated, that means blood-glucose readings from meters can be off by as much as 20 percent and still be valuable.

Q: Wow—isn't that a large number?

A: At first blush, it seems so. But experts nonetheless view SMBG as more accurate than the urine-sugar test, which was previously the only sugar test people could perform at home—and an imprecise one at that.

Q: What is the urine-sugar test and why is it imprecise?

A: The urine-sugar test can detect above-normal blood-sugar levels that occurred a few hours earlier, but it can't give an up-to-the-minute measurement of *blood* sugar, simply because it doesn't test the blood. Obviously, blood tests are a far more accurate source of information about blood-sugar levels.

Q: Going back to glucose meters, what causes a 20 percent error rate?

A: Many things. Sometimes it's a matter of improper technique with the lancet or the meter itself. Mishandling the meter (such as dropping it or leaving it in a hot car) can cause it to malfunction. Improper storage of test strips (exposing them to intense sun or moisture) can lead to a faulty reading.

Another chunk of the blame for misreadings and errors can be put on the quality of instruction that people receive.

Q: What do you mean? Is there a problem with instruction?

A: A report in *Medical World News* says many people with diabetes aren't being taught how to use meters properly—that is, if they are getting any instruction at all. This warning was delivered in 1991 by an advocacy panel of health professionals, consumers, researchers and manufacturers known as the National Steering Committee for Quality Assurance in Capillary Blood Glucose Monitoring (whew!). The panel "implored" physicians, meter manufacturers and other health-care professionals "to improve the way self-monitoring is taught and evaluated," in the words of the report. The committee's research found that "many monitoring errors result from improper training, misunderstanding of instructional materials and bad habits developed over long periods of unsupervised self-monitoring."

And no wonder such problems arose: A two-year scrutiny of diabetes educators by the Food and Drug Administration (FDA) found that the people providing the training didn't understand self-monitoring themselves!

Q: That's incredible! Are you saying that my doctor doesn't know how to use a glucose meter?

A: We can't speak for the skill of any particular health-care practitioner. But we can report that the Food and Drug Administration examined the skills of trainers—people who instruct consumers in meter use—in both medical offices and retail pharmacies. According to the article in *Medical World News*, the average score of office-based trainers was 63 percent and the average score of pharmacy-based trainers was 81 percent—and this on "simple questions that a typical person with diabetes might ask on the use of the meter." If they were receiving report cards, the office-based trainers would bring home a D and the drugstore trainers a B!

When the trainers were asked to take readings on a meter they were familiar with, 43 percent of the blood-glucose levels obtained were outside the acceptable 20 percent deviation. (Another D on the report card!)

Q: All this is rather alarming. What else did the report find?

A: As for the people with diabetes, the FDA found that 37 percent had taught themselves to use their glucose meters. Many learned their testing skills by means of instructional material that the FDA found inadequate.

Accuracy of blood tests is important to all people with diabetes, but particularly for those who follow a regimen of tight control. That's because those folks have a two- to three-times greater risk of developing hypoglycemia—dangerously low blood-sugar levels—than patients on conventional insulin therapy. Some experts postulate that incorrect insulin dosing as a result of monitoring errors may be one reason hypoglycemia is so common.

Q: In light of these problems, what can people with diabetes do to protect themselves?

A: We don't mean to depress you, although certainly this information raises some depressing issues about the fundamental quality of medical instruction. The message here for all people who practice self-monitoring is clear: Be an informed consumer! Get one-on-one training in meter use, perhaps from two or more people. Ask questions if you get conflicting or inconsistent advice.

Q: Are there other self-care tests I should know about?

A: Yes. Besides blood-glucose tests and urine-sugar tests, there is the urine-ketone test (also known as the urine-acetone test, as ketones are sometimes called acetones).

Q: What does the urine-ketone test do?

A: It detects the presence of ketones, or toxins, in the blood. Ketones are formed when fat instead of glucose is burned for energy, which happens when there is no insulin in the blood. People with type-I diabetes use the urine-ketone test to check for the life-threatening condition *ketoacidosis*, or diabetic coma.

Q: Any other tests?

A: There are several other tests that we talk about later in this chapter—ones that, for the time being, must be done in a doctor's office, laboratory or hospital.

Whatever the form, self-testing is only one player on the diabetes self-care team. Another major player is nutrition—the foods we eat.

NUTRITION

Q: Why is nutrition so important?

A: Because diabetes is basically a misfunction in the body's ability to use food as energy, food is an important part of the treatment plan. The kinds of foods a person with diabetes eats, for example, will influence the course of the disease.

Q: So you're talking about diet here?

A: Diet or, as it is also called, the eating plan. No two ways about it: Diet is crucial in the treatment and management of diabetes. That's why people first diagnosed with diabetes are often referred to a dietitian for assistance in analyzing their eating habits and forging better eating plans.

Q: Will a new eating plan call for major changes in the way I eat—restricting certain foods, for instance?

A: It will be necessary to eat well, following sound nutritional principles. You'll have to make some adjustments, perhaps in how much you eat, perhaps in how often, perhaps in what you eat. Whether or not this is a major change depends upon how you've been eating in the past—something we can't tell from where we're sitting.

The *Joslin Diabetes Manual* neatly summarizes the situation: "While some people with diabetes do have to make major diet restrictions, what most lose is the right to overeat or make poor food choices."

Q: What are the proper food choices?

A: Evidence from numerous recent studies documents the importance of a high-fiber, high-complex-carbohydrate diet in improving glucose metabolism. This is a relatively recent change—one that began in 1979 and continued into the mid-1980s as the American Diabetes Association revised its nutritional guidelines to reflect changing research findings. Before then, doctors had always steered their patients toward a low-carbohydrate diet.

As you know, food consists of three nutrients: proteins, fats and carbohydrates. Proteins are used to refurbish the body, replacing worn-out cells with vigorous new ones. Fats are a semipermanent form of nutrient storage. You might envision them as an emergency or backup fuel system.

But when it comes to keeping the body running (or walking or talking), carbohydrates are the real workhorses of the nutrient family. During digestion, carbohydrates are converted either into glucose or glycogen. Glucose is used for immediate energy. Glycogen is glucose in temporary storage, poised and ready to be retrieved at precisely the moment the body calls for energy.

Q: How much of each—proteins, fats and carbohydrates—is necessary?

A: The American Diabetes Association's nutritional guidelines suggest that proteins should account for only 15 to 20 percent of total calories (an even lower amount is suggested for some people with diabetic nephropathy, a form of kidney disease that we discussed in Chapter 4). Fats should account for less than 30 percent and carbohydrates for 55 to 60 percent. Fiber should range from 25 (for women) to 40 grams (for men) a day.

Q: **Wait a minute—how does this diet differ from the one someone without diabetes would follow?**

A: It doesn't, in fact. The high-fiber, high-carbohydrate "diabetic diet" is the same eating plan that is now recommended for the U.S. population in general. Clearly, the ABCs of good eating apply to everyone—with diabetes or not. For people with families, this is good news: It means a healthy diabetic meal is one that the rest of the family can share.

Q: **Must people with type-I and type-II diabetes eat different foods from one another?**

A: An excellent question. As we said, the basic nutritional principles apply to all, so the foods remain the same. However, the goals of diet therapy differ.

People with type-I diabetes follow a simple formula: Eating increases blood sugar; exercise and insulin lower blood sugar. For that reason, people with type-I diabetes are very concerned with the timing of their meals. Meals and snacks must be coordinated with insulin injections and exercise so that blood sugar always remains within target levels.

People with type-II diabetes must remember that eating increases blood sugar, and that consuming a lot of calories at one time can overwhelm the body's limited ability to use insulin efficiently. This limited ability, or insulin resistance, seems to be triggered or intensified by obesity. As most people with type-II diabetes are overweight, their diet goals center on reducing food consumption (which reduces insulin demands on the body) and losing weight (which enables what insulin is present to operate more efficiently).

Since food intake affects blood glucose, both groups (people with type-I and type-II diabetes) should take care not to make any major changes in their diets without consulting their physicians.

Q: Are fats particularly problematic for people with type-II diabetes?

A: Fats are a problem for most Americans, not just people with diabetes, and the recommendation to lower fat to less than 30 percent applies to all people. High levels of dietary fat have been shown to increase the risk of cardiovascular disease—primarily through the effects of fats (known as cholesterol and triglycerides) in the blood.

On top of this, fat is just plain fattening! One gram of fat provides nine calories, but one gram of protein or carbohydrate provides only four calories. That means that, gram for gram, table sugar, as a carbohydrate, has fewer calories than fat! Since many people with diabetes are overweight, reducing fat consumption is the quickest way to begin cutting calories.

Fat comes in three forms—saturated, polyunsaturated and monounsaturated—and the American Diabetes Association recommends that people with diabetes eat some of all three, with the smallest amount being saturated fat.

Q: Why is that?

A: Let's look at where fats are found. Saturated fats come from meat and dairy products, although certain tropical oils (cocoa butter and coconut, palm and palm-kernel oils) are also highly saturated.

Polyunsaturated fats come from vegetable oils, including corn, cottonseed, safflower, soybean and sunflower. Monounsaturated fats are found in olive and canola oils and in avocados. Both polyunsaturated and monounsaturated fats are liquid at room temperature, and they appear to lower cholesterol when they replace saturated fats in the diet.

Q: And lowering cholesterol is a good thing, right?

A: For someone with diabetes, yes.

Years ago, diabetes management revolved simply

around glycemic control. Now physicians know that control of fats, or lipid levels, in the blood is just as important. A high cholesterol level is a major risk factor for atherosclerosis, and blood-fat levels tend to be higher in people with diabetes than in people without the disease.

In particular, people with diabetes tend to have higher levels of low-density lipoprotein (LDL), a substance that some call the "bad cholesterol" because it aids in the deposit of fats on artery and cell walls. In addition, people with diabetes tend to have lower levels of the "good cholesterol," or high-density lipoprotein (HDL), the substance that draws excess cholesterol out of the body. Triglycerides, another form of fat implicated in heart disease (sometimes known as **VLDL**, or very-low-density lipoprotein), are also higher than normal in people with diabetes.

Q: Are people with diabetes more likely to develop high cholesterol levels?

A: For reasons yet unknown, high blood sugar tends to increase cholesterol levels in the blood. Therefore, both type-I and type-II diabetes cause higher cholesterol levels if blood-sugar levels are poorly controlled. For example, extremely high levels of the triglyceride VLDL are commonly found in people experiencing diabetic ketoacidosis.

Q: So lowering blood sugar can lower cholesterol and triglycerides?

A: Yes, it appears that the key to low levels of LDL cholesterol and triglycerides and high levels of HDL, the good cholesterol, lies in glycemic control. In a nutshell, that means carefully managing your disease, by using an eating plan, insulin or oral agent, weight loss, exercise, or (most likely) some combination of these.

Q: So you're saying I should reduce my cholesterol?

A: If you already have high LDL and triglyceride levels, your risk for heart disease increases with each additional lifestyle risk, such as obesity, inactivity, high blood pressure and tobacco use. That's because high fat levels, arterial-wall changes, insulin levels, hypertension and obesity are all factors that combine to accelerate arteriosclerosis in diabetic patients. Changing your diet to lower cholesterol can reduce the risk of heart disease. Evidence suggests that for every 1 percent reduction in blood-cholesterol level, there is a 2 percent reduction in coronary-artery disease.

Q: What if my cholesterol levels aren't really high, merely borderline—is that a problem?

A: Total serum-cholesterol levels (the overall amount of cholesterol in the blood) and LDL-cholesterol levels that are considered borderline for nondiabetic persons are probably of concern in those with diabetes.

Q: What does all this mean? What levels should I strive for?

A: As usual, specific goals vary from person to person; your doctor can help you set precise parameters. But to give you a snapshot of what works for some, here's a list of management goals set by the University of Kentucky Metabolic Research Group, in Lexington, for its adult patients:
- Fasting plasma glucose less than 150 mg/dl
- Total serum cholesterol less than 200 mg/dl
- Fasting serum triglycerides less than 250 mg/dl
- LDL cholesterol less than 130 mg/dl
- HDL cholesterol: over 45 mg/dl in men, over 55 mg/dl in women
- Reaching desirable body weight

Q: So how can I lower my cholesterol levels?

A: One way is to remove the source of cholesterol in your diet by replacing foods that harbor fats with fiber-rich carbohydrates. According to the American Diabetes Association, for a person with diabetes, 55 to 60 percent of daily calories should be derived from carbohydrates. Your physician may quote different figures; we've seen the range as low as 40 to 60 and as high as 60 to 70.

Q: But aren't there differences among carbohydrates?

A: Yes. Carbohydrates come in two forms: simple and complex.

Q: What's a simple carbohydrate?

A: It's one that can be quickly converted into glucose. It also causes a swift rise in blood-glucose levels. Simple carbohydrates are often called simple sugars. They include soft drinks, candy and sugars (table or granulated sugar, brown sugar, molasses and so forth).

Q: I suppose that if I'm concerned about my blood-sugar levels, I should leave sugar out of my diet, right?

A: Not necessarily. For many people this may come as a surprise: Sugar (in moderation) is not taboo. Today's research shows that sugar intake by itself doesn't govern blood-glucose levels. For example, one recent study found that people with type-I diabetes could eat two sugar-laden snacks a day (snacks like brownies and ice cream) with no effect on glycemic control! And the American Diabetes Association has given the thumbs up on a teaspoon of sugar, honey, molasses, or other sweetener per food serving. That's twice the amount of sugar once recommended.

In the eyes of many experts, sugar isn't the real culprit behind diabetic complications, so concerns over sugar intake shouldn't overshadow the real dietary concern—high levels of fat in the diet and a high caloric intake.

Q: **What about artificial sweeteners— are they okay to use?**

A: Saccharin and aspartame are valid substitutes for sugar. Unlike sugar, saccharin is calorie-free. Aspartame contains so few calories per serving that no one counts them.

So, as you see, simple carbohydrates, or simple sugars, can have a place in a meal plan, as long as the person with diabetes realizes that sugar offers only empty calories—not exactly helpful if he is trying to lose weight. Nor is sugar recommended if the person's diabetes is not well controlled.

Q: **Okay—so simple carbohydrates are primarily sugars. What are complex carbohydrates?**

A: Because their cellular structure is more complex, these carbohydrates take longer to be broken down into glucose and absorbed into the bloodstream. Thus, complex carbohydrates don't increase blood-sugar levels as rapidly as simple carbohydrates. Complex carbohydrates include legumes (like beans and peas), grains (like rice), bread, pasta, fruits and starchy vegetables.

The best complex carbohydrates, according to recent research, are those that contain a lot of fiber.

Q: **Fiber—that's plant material, right?**

A: Yes. Fiber is the indigestible material in grains, vegetables and fruits. Fiber can slow the speed at which carbohydrates are absorbed and converted into blood glucose.

The recommendation is that people with diabetes increase their consumption of fiber to 25 grams of fiber for every 1,000 calories. Put another way, that's an average of 40 grams a day for men and 25 grams a day for women. Unfortunately, the average American eats only 11 to 23 grams of fiber daily —meaning that some folks need to double or triple their fiber consumption.

Fiber comes in two forms: insoluble and soluble.

Q: What's the difference between the two?

A: As its name implies, insoluble fiber doesn't dissolve in water. It does absorb water, though, and helps escort foods more quickly through the intestinal system. Foods that contain insoluble fiber include wheat bran, such as that found in whole-grain breads, and certain vegetables and fruits (particularly apple skin, raw carrots and beets).

In contrast, soluble fibers dissolve in water, turning into a thick, gelatinous mass that slows down the rate of glucose absorption. Soluble fibers are helpful for people with diabetes because they help prevent a sharp rise in blood sugar immediately after eating. Foods high in soluble fiber include oat bran, legumes (such as navy, lima and kidney beans), corn, apples and oranges.

The general recommendation is that fiber intake should be increased gradually, perhaps by adding one fiber-rich food per week and including a fiber in every meal, to give the body time to adapt and prevent excessive gas production, a common side effect of added fiber.

Q: What does fiber do?

A: As we mentioned, it slows the speed at which carbohydrates are converted into glucose. And when people with diabetes increase fiber-rich foods and decrease fat-laden ones, they can reduce cholesterol levels and triglyceride levels, at least according to the results of studies at the University of Kentucky. In these studies, people with diabetes followed a diet of 55 to 60 percent carbohydrates and 25 grams of fiber per 1,000 calories. Blood cholesterol fell 15 to 20 percent and triglycerides dipped 40 percent. Researchers believe that such results clinch the argument on the value of high-fiber, high-carbohydrate eating plans.

Just as diet lowers blood sugar, it lowers insulin requirements. People with diabetes may be able to decrease their insulin doses about 10 percent; people with type II may be able to reduce the dose of any oral agent by one-third to one-half.

And because high-fiber foods are very filling and low in fat, they can help people lose weight.

Q: **You've been talking about a high-carbohydrate diet. But I've heard that a low-carbohydrate diet is the best one for diabetes. What gives?**

A: The medical profession is rarely unanimous on any issue, and this one is no exception. A few physicians and dietitians insist that a low-carbohydrate diet is better for some people with type-II diabetes. Richard K. Bernstein, M.D., writing in *Diabetes Type II* (New York: Prentice Hall, 1990), discusses his self-professed "unconventional approach" to diet and diabetes treatment. When it comes to carbohydrates, he recommends that people with type-II diabetes eat only 30 grams a day—equivalent to 2½ slices of white, rye or whole-wheat bread.

Q: **Why such a small amount of carbohydrate?**

A: Bernstein argues that a high-carbohydrate meal makes it impossible to attain normal blood-sugar levels for several hours after eating, and he strives to keep blood-sugar levels normal at all points in the day. (In contrast, most mainstream doctors expect and accept a higher postprandial, or after-meal, blood-sugar reading.)

Under Bernstein's plan, verboten foods include simple sugars, cereals, bread and flour products, rice, certain cooked vegetables (carrots, potatoes, corn, beets, tomatoes) and just about all foods found on the shelves of the average health-food store. His approved foods are grouped under the heading "So What's Left to Eat?" and include most vegetables; meat, fish, fowl, eggs; most cheeses; nuts; and soy products.

He's certainly not the only person in the medical profession who has disputed findings that high-carbohydrate diets lower triglycerides and increase HDL cholesterol. Ann M. Coulston, M.S., R.D., a research dietitian at the Stanford University School of Medicine, claims that when her research group compared the results of people on diets composed of 40 percent versus 60 percent carbohydrates, they found no differences in fasting plasma glucose or in insulin needs.

If you have type-II diabetes and have difficulty digesting high-fiber carbohydrates, or if a high-fiber, high-carbohydrate diet doesn't seem to control your blood sugar, then you might wish to read and discuss Bernstein's book with your health-care practitioner.

Q: These conflicting opinions are very disorienting. How do I decide what treatment course to follow?

A: You can't make the decision alone—you must make it in conjunction with your health-care practitioner, who is your partner in health care. Discuss the issue with your physician. It's always essential for any person with diabetes, as a medical consumer, to delve into issues and discuss them with her doctor. The moral is: Speak up!

Q: Okay, let's say my doctor and I figure out the right balance of protein, fat, carbohydrates and fiber. What's the next step?

A: Decide *how much* to eat. This is crucial for people with type-I diabetes, because the projected size of their meals determines insulin doses. Once insulin is injected, people with diabetes can't eat more or less than planned without throwing blood sugar out of whack.

Q: What about those of us with type-II diabetes?

A: As you may recall from our discussion of type-II diabetes, part of the treatment is reducing food intake —eating less, in effect. The reason is simple: The more food you eat, the greater the demand for insulin.

The amount you need to eat depends upon your age, height, sex and the amount of exercise you get. Your health-care practitioner or a dietitian can help you map out the appropriate number of calories you need each day.

You need to be precise about your calorie needs if you must lose weight or if you are concerned about gaining it— because too much food causes too many pounds. As the *Joslin Diabetes Manual* explains it, "Obese people often look for excuses beyond their control, such as a 'glandular condition' or 'stress,' but the basic reason that they are over-weight is that they have eaten more calories than they need."

Q: Is there anything else people with diabetes need to keep in mind?

A: Yes, and that's the frequency of meals. Generally the experts agree that "small feedings"—three or four small meals a day—are better than one large daily meal.

Doctors recommend that people using insulin schedule their meals so that they eat something—if only a snack—at peak insulin times. People with type-II diabetes who don't use insulin are encouraged to spread out their caloric consumption into three meals and several snacks, so that they aren't calling on their pancreas to produce large amounts of insulin to cope with one or two large meals.

And an article in the *New England Journal of Medicine* suggests another reason for spreading out caloric consumption: People who eat frequent small meals (particularly those high in soluble fiber, which prolongs absorption time) may be less likely to experience those higher levels of cholesterol and triglycerides that accompany diabetes.

Q: Do all complex carbohydrates slow increases in blood glucose?

A: As studies were done on various foods and their effects on blood sugar, researchers discovered that different carbohydrates break down at different rates. The carbohydrates in a potato, for instance, are converted into glucose more quickly than the carbohydrates in rice.

From this observation about the differing glycemic effects of food came a rather controversial concept called the **glycemic index**.

Q: Just what does this glycemic index do?

A: The glycemic index was developed by scientists at the University of Toronto to calculate how foods affect blood-glucose levels. For example, in a laboratory setting, both honey and cooked carrots raised blood-sugar levels 80 to 90 percent as high as straight glucose did, while lentils and kidney beans raised blood sugar a mere 20 to 29 percent as high as glucose did. Taking this data, scientists assigned a different glycemic value to a whole host of foods. The glycemic index was useful in scientific measurements, and the hope was that it might be useful to people with diabetes—the idea being that by knowing the glycemic value of certain foods, people would eat those foods less likely to raise blood glucose.

Q: The glycemic index sounds rather useful. Why is it controversial?

A: The biggest reason is that in real life, a food's glycemic index is not a fixed number. It changes depending on whether the food is cooked, how it's cooked, how long it's cooked, and what other foods are eaten along with it. For that reason and others, experts don't see the glycemic index as a helpful tool for day-to-day meal planning.

Q: Is there anything that can make meal planning simpler?

A: To help people with diabetes wade through the meal-planning waters, the American Diabetes Association and the American Dietetic Association developed the exchange system.

Q: What's this?

A: Here's how it works: Under this system, foods are grouped into six categories: bread and starch, vegetables, fruit, milk, meat, and fat. The foods in each category, when eaten in the portions indicated, have the same number of calories and the same nutritional value. For instance, under the bread and starch category, one-third of a cup of vegetarian baked beans has the same number of calories as one slice of raisin bread.

You can see how this makes calorie counting and meal planning less painful—all the calorie-counting footwork has been done. The exchange system helps people accurately coordinate their insulin doses with the amount of food they eat. It also helps other people set up a plan to lose weight. As long as they use the specified portions, people can exchange one food under a heading with another food from that same group, knowing that both foods have the same number of calories and the same nutritional content.

Q: Speaking of nutritional content, what's the official stand on caffeine—is it something people with diabetes must avoid?

A: The amount of caffeine in a couple of cups of coffee or tea or in several soft drinks isn't going to affect diabetes control. For that reason, most doctors say that coffee and tea are fine in the diet.

However, as with any kind of food product, moderation is the key. Very large amounts of caffeine (5 to 10 cups of coffee a day) may raise blood sugar. Furthermore, the adverse effects of too much caffeine are often confused with signs of an insulin reaction, or vice versa: anxiety, trembling and irritability.

Q: Can people with diabetes drink alcohol?

A: Most can—in moderation, of course. Excessive drinking, however, is likely to wreak havoc with a blood-glucose level, sending it spiraling downward by interfering with the way the liver processes glycogen.

In addition, diabetic drugs known as oral hypoglycemic agents (especially first-generation oral agents—see Chapter 3) may interact with alcohol, causing facial flushing, severe headaches or dizziness. If that happens, you could ask your doctor to put you on a different oral agent. The new drug might not interact with alcohol but then again it might— doctors find it impossible to predict who will be affected by which drug. As a result, some people using oral agents find it less aggravating not to drink at all.

If you choose to have an occasional drink (and many people with diabetes do), be aware that alcohol contains empty calories—they have no nutritional value. Those calories must be accounted for when someone is trying to lose or maintain weight.

Q: Do dietary supplements have a role in diabetes care? For instance, do people with diabetes need extra vitamins?

A: Many practitioners recommend a daily multivitamin-mineral supplement, in part because they believe that frequent urination (a hallmark of high blood-sugar levels) may discharge needed nutrients, and in part because they worry that a high-fiber, high-carbohydrate diet may lead to vitamin and mineral binding, which is caused when a food prevents a vitamin or mineral from being absorbed during digestion.

In general, the mainstream medical profession is not enthusiastic about large doses of vitamins for anyone, let alone people with diabetes. It has been noted that large doses of vitamin C can lead to unreliable readings of urine-sugar tests—something to keep in mind if you plan to use that test.

Q: What about fish-oil supplements?

A: Eating fish can help prevent coronary-heart disease by lowering cholesterol levels, according to numerous studies. However, while fish-oil supplements—specifically omega-3—may help control cholesterol, studies show that they increase blood-sugar levels. Over the long haul, the increased blood-sugar levels would erase any benefit of the fish oil on cardiovascular disease.

Today, experts recommend that people with diabetes eat fish, but they advise staying away from fish-oil supplements.

Q: I've heard that cinnamon can improve blood sugar. Can you tell me more?

A: When Richard Anderson, a researcher with the U.S. Department of Agriculture, heard several stories of people using a daily sprinkle of cinnamon to help control their blood sugar, he decided to test the spice—as well as several others—in test-tube experiments. He found that even tiny amounts of cinnamon extract were nine times better than other spices at reducing the amount of insulin needed to break down glucose. Because his research was done strictly in test tubes, he didn't test cinnamon's effect on people or animals. But it sure sounds like a tasty way to keep glucose in line.

Q: If a spice might reduce blood sugar, might the same be possible for herbs? Are there any herbal approaches to treating diabetes?

A: Much of the use of plant treatments for diabetes (as well as the research into their effectiveness) is done overseas in Britain and other areas of Europe, and in Asia, where **homeopathic** and **herbal medicine** play a greater role in health care than in the United States. (Homeopathic medicine treats illnesses by using safe, natural medicines that stimulate a person's own healing powers while avoiding harmful side effects. Herbal medicine is a healing art that uses plants to prevent and cure illnesses.)

For those who would like to read more about this topic, we suggest a visit to a local hospital library for a copy of an article in the September 1989 issue of *Diabetes Care*. This article discussed plant treatments in great detail, noting that only a small number of the over 400 traditional plant treatments for diabetes have yet been scientifically and medically evaluated. The authors state that a plant-based substitute for insulin is unlikely to be found, but, they wrote, "traditional treatments may provide valuable clues for the development of new oral hypoglycemic agents and simple dietary adjuncts."

Q: For example?

A: Two plants that have been found to lower blood glucose in people with type-II diabetes during clinical trials are *Coccinia indica* (ivy gourd) and *Momordica charantia* (karela). Both reduced blood-glucose levels by about 20 percent shortly after test subjects with diabetes took them, and both improved overall glycemic control when they were used for several months. Researchers postulate that these plants contain substances that may lead to the development of new drugs.

Some plants mentioned in the *Diabetes Care* article were thought to produce a beneficial effect in large part because they were high in fiber. Other plants reduced blood glucose, but at a cost—they also had unhealthy toxic effects.

Q: What about vegetarianism? Is it healthy?

A: A carefully planned vegetarian diet can be very healthy. Long-term retrospective studies of vegetarians find that they live longer and healthier lives than their peers eating the typical American high-protein, high-fat diet. For one thing, vegetarians are less likely to develop heart disease. Legumes (beans and peas), which are staples of vegetarian eating plans, are high in fiber and so are thought to help lower serum-cholesterol levels.

The thing to remember is that there are lots of different foods in the world and lots of opportunities to mix them in creative, satisfying and nutritional combinations. Of course, a "good" diet or meal plan is not just one that is nutritionally sound—it has to be one that the person with diabetes will eat! In other words, it has to be appetizing to the individual palate. It can—and should—take into account ethnic preferences.

Q: What do you mean by "ethnic preferences"?

A: Different ethnic groups historically tend to prefer different types of food. For instance, a healthy lunch for a Caucasian may include a sandwich with whole-wheat bread. A sandwich probably wouldn't appeal to a Navajo, who comes from a culture that eats very little wheat flour— but a mutton, bean and vegetable stew with a corn tortilla might hit the spot. Since diabetes strikes a disproportionate share of some minority groups in this country, people with diabetes shouldn't hesitate to develop (or ask a dietitian to locate) recipes that they find palatable.

Q: What else can you tell me about diet?

A: It's not our goal to be encyclopedic about nutrition, but we do wish to impress upon you the effect on blood sugar of the foods you choose to eat. There are plenty of sources of more information on fats and carbohydrates (some listed at the end of this chapter). If you're interested, search these out. The more information you have about your disease, the wiser a medical consumer you'll become, and the better a partner you'll be in your health care.

Q: Whew—let's say I've mastered nutrition. Now I can put up my feet and relax for a while, right?

A: Not so fast! You'd probably be better off slipping on a pair of walking shoes and heading out for a brisk 20-minute jaunt in the fresh air, because exercise is the third crucial element in the treatment of diabetes.

EXERCISE

Q: What does exercise do?

A: Exercise does many things—it improves one's state of mind, builds muscle tone and speeds the process of losing weight. Most of all for people with diabetes, it lowers blood sugar by making tissues more sensitive to insulin. Twenty minutes of fast walking, for instance, may bring blood glucose down 20 mg/dl.

A person with diabetes who is out of shape or just plain new to an exercise regimen may need to check with a health-care practitioner before launching into an exercise program. A physician can give him details about the optimum heartbeat rate for someone his age, weight and overall physical condition. Since exercise lowers blood sugar, people with type-I diabetes will initially need medical assistance in determining how to adjust food intake and insulin doses on their new exercise plans. In fact, people who are insulin-dependent— or those with type-II diabetes who are on oral agents—need to exercise a few precautions before exercising their limbs.

Q: What precautions are these?

A: They may need to eat before, during or after exercising to compensate for the anticipated drop in blood sugar. Many exercisers who have diabetes carry a small sugary snack in case blood-sugar levels fall too low. If they're insulin-dependent and exercise vigorously, they should inform the people they exercise with and teach them about the symptoms of hypoglycemia (low blood sugar). Wearing a bracelet or necklace or carrying a wallet card that identifies the exerciser as insulin-dependent is an extra measure of precaution.

Q: What types of exercise are best?

A: Most authorities in the field recommend that a three-times-a-week program of walking, swimming, jogging, bicycling, aerobics, rowing, hiking, cross-country skiing—whatever a person can handle, as long as it gets her heart pumping for 20 to 30 minutes and makes her work up a sweat. These exercises, called **aerobic exercises**, build cardiovascular fitness.

Exercise buffs will tell you that it's important to warm up before exercising and to cool down afterward. Look for flexibility exercises—stretching and bending—to help you loosen up your joints and prepare your muscles for the work ahead. Flexibility exercises reduce the chance of injuring muscles.

Q: You mentioned exercising three times a week. Why does it have to be that often?

A: Frequent exercise is essential because the benefit of exercise on insulin efficiency does not last very long. People who are trying to lose weight might do well to remember that the more often they exercise, the more calories they burn. Exercising three or more times a week can help people lose weight faster.

Q: So exercise can be very helpful?

A: Extremely beneficial for many people with diabetes— and perhaps even crucial for people who have a family history of diabetes but who have not yet developed the disease.

Q: Why is that?

A: Research from Harvard Medical School in Boston has found that regular vigorous exercise—the kind that induces a sweat—may protect people against developing diabetes. In their study of 87,253 women from 1980 to 1988, the researchers found that, compared with women who did not exercise, women who exercised vigorously at least once a week lowered by one-third the risk of developing type-II diabetes.

Q: What kind of vigorous exercise?

A: Brisk walking, playing tennis, jogging, swimming, hiking, bicycling and the like. *Strenuous* is another word researchers use to describe activities that make you sweat.

Even a simple routine of "power" walking or swimming several days a week can help. And there's more good news— the Harvard study showed the benefit of exercise held true whether the women were obese, moderately overweight or not overweight, and was beneficial regardless of family history of diabetes.

Q: What about men?

A: Recent research has since confirmed the same phenomenon in men. One study, reported in the

Journal of the American Medical Association in 1992, found that the more frequently the men exercised, the less likely they were to develop type-II diabetes, even in the face of other risk factors, such as smoking, high blood pressure and obesity! Men who worked up a sweat five or more times a week had 42 percent less risk of developing diabetes than those who exercised less than once a week. Men who worked out two to four times per week reduced the risk 38 percent, and those who broke a sweat once a week reduced the risk 23 percent.

Q: Can anyone with diabetes exercise?

A: A good question. In theory, exercise is good for everyone. It gets the circulation going, lowers blood sugar, increases muscle tone, guards against osteoporosis in women and lowers the risk of heart disease. In people with type-II diabetes, exercise in combination with a well-crafted meal plan can burn off unwanted fat while increasing the body's sensitivity to insulin.

There are some caveats, however. Once someone is relying on insulin (and that includes many people with type-II diabetes as well as most who have type I), exercise takes on a different dimension. Exercise has to be planned for, and insulin doses adjusted as appropriate. Insulin users should not exercise when they are ill, even if it's something as minor as a cold or flu. Blood-sugar levels are difficult enough to control during illness without adding another variable in the form of exercise.

Nor should someone with diabetes exercise on his feet when he has a foot injury. Exercise might exacerbate a blister, bruise or cut, resulting in an infection or an ulcer.

Sad to say, too, that some people with diabetes can't exercise because their disease has already progressed too far.

Q: In what way?

A: In particular, regular physical activity may not be possible for people who have developed severe diabetic complications. One study that looked at 837 hospitalized people with insulin-treated type-II diabetes found that 69 percent had at least one complication that precluded vigorous exercise or demanded special precautionary measures if exercise was to be attempted. Granted, those folks were hospitalized and so had a more severe form of diabetes than many of their peers. But the lesson is clear: People with diabetes must begin exercise programs as early in the course of their disease as possible, before it's too late to reap exercise's many benefits.

On the whole, though, exercise is pretty amazing stuff, apparently preventing the development of type-II diabetes and helping those who already have the disease to bring their blood sugar into control. Perhaps we might suggest (with tongue only slightly in cheek) that people who are at risk of developing diabetes run, not walk, to their doctor's office to discuss setting up an exercise regimen.

Which brings us to a related area of self-care—the proper care of your feet.

FOOT CARE

Q: What do you mean by proper foot care?

A: For starters, examine your feet every day for even minor problems, such as cuts, corns, bruises and blisters. If undetected, any one of these seemingly simple problems can lead to a major infection and, if you're very unlucky, gangrene. Diabetic foot disease is the cause of 20 percent of hospitalizations for people with diabetes and, as we mentioned in Chapter 4, diabetes-related amputations account for half of all nontrauma-associated amputations performed in the United States. Fortunately, there are ways to prevent yourself from becoming one of those statistics. Here's how:

- Inspect and wash your feet daily in warm (not hot) water; blot to dry, and do not rub between the toes. Use a moisturizing cream (but not between the toes).
- Change shoes twice daily. Wear leather shoes with large toe boxes, such as soft leather jogging shoes.
- Wear clean cotton or wool socks that are the proper size for your feet.
- Don't use hot-water bottles, heating pads or heat lamps near your feet.
- Don't cross your legs when sitting (it reduces circulation in the legs) and don't wear garters.
- Don't cut your toenails—file them so that they are straight across. Slightly round the corners by filing them diagonally.
- Don't use chemical agents to remove corns or calluses, and don't use inserts or pads without checking with your health-care practitioner.
- Don't wear new shoes for more than an hour at one time until they are broken in, and don't wear shoes without socks.
- Never go barefoot out-of-doors! Sandals and open-toed shoes are invitations to problems.

DENTAL CARE

Q: Are there any other areas of the body that need special attention?

A: Yes, the teeth and gums. Uncontrolled diabetes seems to increase the risk of gum disease (a major cause of tooth loss) and leads to more cavities.

Regular dental self-care (brushing and flossing teeth) and regular dental checkups are important in people with high blood sugar. Watch for the signs of gum disease, which include bleeding or swollen gums, receding gums and loose teeth, and report them to your dentist immediately.

And speaking of the mouth—one thing you should never put in it is a cigarette.

SMOKING

Q: Are you telling me to give up smoking?

A: No, that's something you should tell yourself. Everyone knows that cigarette smoking increases the risk
of heart disease and lung cancer. Smoking definitely has
those negative impacts on people with diabetes—and it tacks
on others.

Q: Such as?

A: Studies suggest that insulin users who smoke require
15 to 20 percent more insulin than nonsmokers. But
the biggest reason to give up smoking is that it increases the
risk of diabetes-related complications, such as cardiovascular
and kidney disease, by accelerating small-blood-vessel damage.
People with diabetes already have higher rates of cardiovascular and kidney complications—why compound the risk?

Q: Is there anything else I should know about
diabetes self-care?

A: Since you asked, now is the perfect time to look at
some special situations related to diabetes care. Inter-
estingly enough, these pertain to certain times of life: youth
and adolescence, the childbearing years and advanced age.

CHILDREN AND DIABETES

Q: Are the treatment goals of diabetes different
in children?

A: As with adults, the goal is to keep blood sugar within
normal ranges and to prevent the dangerous short-
term complications hypoglycemia and ketoacidosis. And of

course, good exercise and eating habits must be part of the treatment plan.

Q: Can children practice self-care?

A: Once they get to be of school age, yes. They can be taught to recognize the symptoms of hypoglycemia and ketoacidosis, understand the fundamentals of meal planning, and even self-monitor their blood glucose.

Very young children obviously require extra care from Mom and Dad, and even older kids still need supervision to ensure they balance exercise with food intake or that they don't overindulge in sweets with friends. Teenagers, who are often fiercely independent (or try to be), may resent having to practice a somewhat rigid meal and medicine routine. They may try to take shortcuts, such as neglecting their SMBG. However, the hormonal changes of puberty can make blood-sugar levels less predictable, meaning SMBG is required more often rather than less. Parents and doctors may find that they may have to work out some type of compromise with teenagers, trading extra control in one area (SMBG, for example) with more flexibility in another (such as type of food eaten).

There are many excellent sources of diabetes information designed just for young people—both children and teenagers —and we list some at the end of this chapter. Use them! And remember, it's never too early to teach self-care—or to practice it.

PREGNANCY AND DIABETES

Q: What about diabetes and pregnancy—what special self-care steps are involved here?

A: Women with diabetes who plan to become pregnant should first get blood-sugar levels under control, using the strategies we've discussed in this book. Well-managed diabetes reduces the risk of complications during pregnancy, but pregnancy requires extra effort and attention to blood sugar, caloric intake, nutritional balance and exercise. Even with extra care there are potential problems, such as premature birth, an abnormally large baby, difficult birth, or an infant born with respiratory problems, low blood calcium, jaundice or an infection.

The insulin doses and food required to control diabetes change during pregnancy: A woman may need close to three times more insulin by the time she is ready to deliver. The goal, as with all insulin therapy, is to keep blood sugar as close to normal ranges as possible. After the pregnancy, the treatment returns to that used before the pregnancy. Women are encouraged to breast-feed their babies (though that may require additional insulin), as it's good for the health of both mother and child.

Q: What about self-care issues related to gestational diabetes?

A: As you may recall, gestational diabetes is any type of diabetes that first appears during pregnancy. In 95 percent of the cases, it disappears after childbirth.

Gestational-diabetes symptoms are generally mild and not life threatening to the women. The condition, however, can pose problems for their infants, including hypoglycemia and respiratory distress. Most women are able to control gestational diabetes through diet and exercise, although a few go on to use human insulin. (Oral agents cannot be used during pregnancy.) Self-monitoring of blood glucose is mandatory.

All women with diabetes can expect to undergo additional tests during the course of pregnancy.

Q: What kinds of tests?

A: They might include fetal tests, such as the **alpha fetoprotein** test, to check for possible spinal defects. **Ultrasound** tests check the health and development of the fetus and estimate its weight and size (information that determines whether the baby can be delivered through the vagina

or if a cesarean delivery may be required). Other tests may include an electrocardiogram to check heart condition, kidney-function tests, urine-ketone tests and frequent eye exams to watch for diabetic retinopathy. Women who have moderate to severe retinopathy may need to be examined as often as once a month, because pregnancy speeds the course of this disease.

On the whole, women with diabetes or gestational diabetes need to get frequent medical attention, with an eye on controlling blood sugar and pregnancy-related complications. Again, turn to the resources section of this book for additional information.

AGING AND DIABETES

Q: Okay, what about an area of concern further along the time line—diabetes and aging?

A: Blood-glucose levels begin to increase in everyone in their 50s and 60s. And while people may not develop diabetes per se, they may develop impaired glucose tolerance (also called glucose intolerance), or slight elevations in blood sugar. This may be a function of aging, and it may be related to insulin resistance associated with being overweight. Either way, even slight increases in blood sugar put people at greater risk of cardiovascular problems, meaning that the elderly need to pay special attention to diet and exercise.

Q: Can anything be done about glucose intolerance?

A: Food may play a role in preventing or slowing its onset. In one recently published study, Dutch researchers found that 60 percent of people aged 64 to 87 who regularly ate fish—usually an ounce a day—were less likely to develop glucose intolerance than people who didn't eat fish.

Q: What about full-fledged diabetes in the elderly. Do the concerns change?

A: Elderly people with diabetes may have difficulty adhering to their regimen for unique reasons. Vision problems or decreased manual dexterity may make it more difficult to use syringes or glucose meters accurately. Exercise plans become more difficult to maintain. Kidney function also declines with age, which means the elderly face a greater risk of kidney complications. Of course, not all older people with diabetes have these problems—many are robust and healthy. But to make the task of self-care easier on the elderly, some doctors recommend more frequent blood tests, a simple meal plan and office visits every three months to check for eye and foot problems.

Q: Speaking of office visits, what kind of care should I expect from my physician?

A: Choosing a doctor is always a personal matter. You want someone who will listen to your opinions and treat you with respect—in short, someone who will treat you as an equal partner in health care.

Whether you choose someone who specializes in diabetes care or someone whose treatment methods lean away from the medical mainstream, this is a decision that only you can make.

However, it's important that your practitioner strive to keep you as healthy as possible. And that means a focus on prevention—prevention of diabetes complications.

Q: Aren't all physicians concerned with prevention?

A: Yes and no. Recent reports suggest that primary-care physicians are not very reliable about performing preventive exams in patients with diabetes. According to a representative from the Centers for Disease Control and Prevention (CDC), self-reports from more than 1,000 primary-care physicians suggest not all doctors are up-to-date on recommended tests and examinations. In addition, the CDC has found that people with type-I diabetes generally receive more preventive services than do those with type II. Apparently, type-II diabetes is still seen as less serious than type-I diabetes—a problem in attitude that we discussed in the opening pages of this book.

Q: **What kind of preventive services are recommended?**

A: They include quarterly blood-pressure measurements, twice-a-year foot examinations, annual exams for diabetic retinopathy, regular inspection of gums and teeth (a relatively new recommendation), and certain tests: the **glycosylated hemoglobin**, urine protein and creatinine clearance tests.

Q: **Could you tell me more about these lab tests?**

A: Sure thing. One of the newest and most important is the glycosylated hemoglobin.

Q: **Glyco . . . what?**

A: The glycosylated hemoglobin test, also called the **hemoglobin A_{1c} test**, measures the number of glucose molecules ("glyco") attached to hemoglobin, a substance within the red blood cells. This gives a reading of the average sugar level over the previous six to eight weeks—in contrast to a blood-glucose test, which gives a reading of blood glucose at only one particular moment in time.

The glycosylated hemoglobin test is one of the most important ways of measuring overall diabetes control. Performed every three months or so, it shows you and your doctor how well your treatment regimen is working by telling where your glucose levels have been, on average, for the last two months. The test also shows if the data gathered from SMBG are reasonably accurate.

Q: Are there any other tests?

A: The following are some of the most common laboratory tests. Certain of these tests should be performed several times a year; others should be done yearly (or less often, depending upon the severity of your disease).

• Cholesterol test (sometimes called a lipid profile). This is actually a series of tests that measure lipids, or fatty substances, in the blood. These tests include 1) total serum cholesterol, 2) HDL cholesterol, and 3) triglycerides. They are performed to determine a person's total cholesterol, LDL cholesterol level and triglyceride levels. High levels of these increase the risk of heart disease and often are signals of inadequate diabetes control, as we mentioned earlier in this chapter.

• Urinalysis. This screens for urinary-tract infections (which, if allowed unchecked, may lead to kidney damage).

• Creatinine clearance. This test measures the filtering capacity of the kidneys, and thus is used to monitor deterioration of the kidneys. It requires a blood test and a ''24-hour urine specimen''—that is, all the urine a person produced in 24 hours.

• Microalbuminuria. This test also reflects early kidney changes and often requires a 24-hour urine collection.

Many other tests may be done depending upon the severity of your disease and may include an electrocardiogram, an angiogram or a thyroid function test. Many of these are geared toward detecting or evaluating a diabetic complication.

Q: You didn't mention a blood-glucose test. Why is that?

A: At first glance, it might seem that a blood-glucose test should be a part of the battery of office tests. In fact, guidelines set by the American College of Physicians in 1990 call for the use of home glucose testing as a substitute for routine testing in a doctor's office.

If you think about it, that makes sense. Since people with diabetes can self-monitor blood glucose with any of the simple home testing kits, why pay for a blood-sugar reading in a doctor's office when it can—and, some say, should—be done at home? Just be sure to bring your notebook with your SMBG results to the doctor's office, so she can see the most recent blood-sugar levels.

Q: It sounds like self-care all boils down to my taking responsibility for the treatment of my disease.

A: In many ways, yes. Although you will work closely with your doctor, it's ultimately up to you to make the commitment to control your disease, instead of letting it control you.

Q: What else can help me in this mission?

A: Keep asking questions—and get answers to them. Here's a list of organizations that can guide you to more sources of information.

American Association of Diabetes Educators
500 N. Michigan Ave., Suite 1400
Chicago, IL 60611
(312) 661-1700

American Diabetes Association, National Center
1660 Duke St.
Alexandria, VA 22314
(800) 232-3472
Local chapters of this organization will be listed in
your phone book.

American Dietetic Association
216 W. Jackson Blvd., Suite 800
Chicago, IL 60606-6995
(312) 899-0040

Juvenile Diabetes Foundation International
432 Park Avenue South
New York, NY 10016-8103
(800) 223-1138
(212) 889-7575

National Diabetes Information Clearinghouse
Box NDIC
9000 Rockville Pike
Bethesda, MD 20892
(301) 468-2162

GLOSSARY

Absorbency: How quickly insulin takes effect.

Acetohexamide: Oral hypoglycemic agent; used to lower blood-sugar levels.

Acetones: See **Ketones.**

Acute: Begins quickly and is intense, then slowing after a short time; sharp or severe.

Adult-onset diabetes: Term once used for **type-II diabetes.**

Aerobic exercise: Steady activity that gets your heart pumping and makes you work up a sweat.

Aldose reductase: Enzyme thought to play a role in triggering diabetes complications.

Aldose reductase inhibitors: Class of drugs that block the action of the enzyme aldose reductase.

Algorithm: A simple mathematical chart that can serve as a guide for determining how many units of insulin to take and when to take them, depending upon blood-sugar level.

Alpha fetoprotein: Test that screens for possible spinal defects in an unborn baby.

Angiogram: X-ray that locates blockages in large blood vessels.

Antigens: Proteins or enzymes capable of stimulating an immune response.

Arteriosclerosis: Hardening of the arteries.

Artery: Blood vessel that carries blood away from the heart.

Atherosclerosis: Form of arteriosclerosis in which inner walls of arteries thicken due to deposits of fat, cholesterol and other substances.

Autoimmune: Term used to describe what happens when the body's immune system attacks itself.

Autonomic neuropathy: Damage to the nerves that control bodily functions like the digestive system, urinary tract and cardiovascular system.

Background retinopathy: Mild, early form of the disease of retinal blood vessels.

Beef-derived insulin: Insulin obtained from the pancreas of a steer.

Beta cells: Cells in the pancreas that produce and secrete insulin into the bloodstream when blood-sugar levels rise.

Blood glucose: Blood sugar. Body's primary source of energy.

Blood-glucose meter: Device to test blood-sugar levels.

Blood pressure: Force of blood against the walls of blood vessels.

Borderline diabetes: Another term for **impaired glucose tolerance.**

Brittle diabetes: Dramatic swings in blood-glucose levels.

Bypass surgery: Method of rerouting blood around obstructions in a blood vessel.

Capillaries: Minute blood vessels that carry blood between the smallest arteries and the smallest veins.

Carbohydrate: One of the three basic sources of energy in food; found in grains, vegetables and fruits.

Cardiac: Pertaining to the heart.

Cardiovascular: Pertaining to the heart and blood vessels.

Cataract: A clouding of the lens of the eye or of its surrounding transparent membrane that obstructs the passage of light.

Catheter: A tubular medical device for insertion into canals, vessels or body cavities usually to allow injection or withdrawal of fluids.

Chlorpropamide: Oral hypoglycemic agent; used to lower blood-sugar levels.

Cholesterol: Fatlike substance that comes from meat and dairy products.

Chronic: Referring to a condition or disease that develops slowly and persists for a long period of time.

Closed-loop pump: Implantable **insulin pump.**

Combination therapy: Treatment of type-II diabetes using a combination of **insulin** and an **oral hypoglycemic agent.**

Complex carbohydrate: Carbohydrate made from more complex chains of sugar that are digested more slowly and raise blood sugar less rapidly than **simple carbohydrate.**

Continuous subcutaneous insulin infusion (CSII): Form of intensive insulin therapy using an **insulin pump.**

Conventional therapy: In diabetes, use of insulin to keep blood-sugar levels within certain target ranges; less stringent than **tight control.**

Dawn phenomenon: Sudden increase in blood sugar that occurs in early morning.

Degree: Intensity of effect or the activity insulin creates.

Diabetes mellitus: Disease resulting from the body's inability to produce or use insulin, resulting in high blood-sugar levels.

Diabetic coma: Another term used for **ketoacidosis,** or dangerously high blood-sugar levels, which can cause coma and death.

Dialysis: Use of a machine to filter wastes from blood after kidneys have failed.

Diet therapy: Use of an eating plan to lower blood sugar.

Duration: The length of time of the effect or the activity insulin creates.

Epinephrine: Naturally occurring hormone that works to keep insulin and sugar levels balanced; also called adrenaline.

Euglycemia: Normal levels of blood sugar.

Fasting: Not eating for three or more hours.

Fasting plasma glucose test: Measurement of blood-sugar level before the first meal of the day, usually 12 hours after eating.

Fat: One of the three basic sources of energy in food; found in dairy products, meat, fish, nuts, oils and some vegetables.

Fiber: Indigestible material in grains, vegetables and fruits; see **insoluble fiber** and **soluble fiber.**

Fructose: Sugar in fruits, vegetables and honey.

Gangrene: Death of body tissues due to a loss of blood supply.

Gestational diabetes: Diabetes that develops or is discovered in a woman during pregnancy.

Glipizide: Oral hypoglycemic agent; used to lower blood-sugar levels.

Glomeruli: Tuftlike structures composed of blood vessels or nerve fibers.

Glucagon: Naturally occurring hormone (produced by the pancreas) that increases blood sugar.

Glucose: Sugar; the body's primary energy source.

Glyburide: Oral hypoglycemic agent; used to lower blood-sugar levels.

Glycemia: Blood-sugar level.

Glycemic: Pertaining to blood-sugar level.

Glycemic control: Overall control of blood sugar.

Glycemic index: Scientific measurement of the effect of different foods on blood-sugar levels.

Glycogen: Storage form of glucose.

Glycosylated hemoglobin: Test that measures the number of glucose molecules attached to hemoglobin, a substance within the red blood cells; used to estimate average blood sugar over the prior two months.

Hemoglobin A$_{1c}$ test: Term sometimes used for the **glycosylated hemoglobin** test.

Hemorrhage: A loss of a large amount of blood in a short period of time, either outside or inside the body.

Herbal medicine: Healing art that uses plants to prevent and cure illnesses.

High blood pressure: Increase in blood pressure above normal levels; also called hypertension.

High-density lipoprotein (HDL): "Good" cholesterol; substance that escorts excess cholesterol out of the body.

Homeopathic medicine: Treats illnesses by using safe, natural medicines that stimulate a person's own healing powers while avoiding harmful side effects.

Human insulin: Insulin manufactured to be chemically identical to the insulin normally produced by the body.

Hypercholesterolemia: High levels of cholesterol in the blood.

Hyperglycemia: High blood-sugar levels.

Hyperinsulinemia: High levels of insulin in the blood.

Hyperlipidemia: High levels of fatty substances in the blood.

Hyperosmolar coma: Dangerous dehydration and/or loss of consciousness caused by high blood-sugar levels; differs chemically from **ketoacidosis.**

Hypertension: High blood pressure.

Hypertriglyceridemia: High levels of triglycerides in the blood.

Hypoglycemia: Low blood sugar.

Hypoglycemic unawareness: Occurs when people with low blood-sugar levels do not experience or detect the warning signals of hypoglycemia.

Iatrogenic: Caused by medical treatment.

Immunosuppressive drugs: Drugs used to stop the immune system from attacking some substance.

Immunotherapy: Method of treatment used to stop the immune system from attacking some substance.

Impaired glucose tolerance (IGT): Blood-sugar levels higher than normal but not high enough to be diagnosed as diabetes.

Implantable pump: A small device inserted under the skin that pumps insulin into the body at specified intervals.

Impotence: Loss of male sexual functioning.

Increased risk for diabetes: Term applied to someone at increased risk of developing diabetes in the future.

Injection site: Area where insulin is injected.

Insoluble fiber: Indigestible material, found in certain grains, vegetables and fruits, that absorbs water but doesn't dissolve in it.

Insulin: Hormone produced in pancreas that enables the body to use sugar for energy.

Insulin allergy: Adverse reaction to insulin.

Insulin-dependent diabetes: Term sometimes used for **type-I diabetes.**

Insulin pen: Device shaped like a pen; used to inject insulin.

Insulin pump: Battery-operated device that pumps insulin into the body at specified intervals.

Insulin reaction: Low blood sugar caused by too much insulin, not enough food or too much exercise.

Insulin resistance: Term applied when insulin is produced by the body but is not being used efficiently.

Insulin shock: Hypoglycemic shock caused by an overdose of insulin, a decreased intake of food, or too much exercise; characterized by trembling, sweating, nervousness, irritability, hunger, hallucination, numbness and pallor.

Intensive therapy: Type of diabetes therapy that strives for tight control of blood-sugar levels within certain narrow targets. Also known as **tight control.**

Intermediate-acting insulin: Insulin that works more quickly than **long-acting insulin** but not as quickly as **short-acting insulin.**

Intraocular lens: Artificial lens implanted in eye.

Islets, or **islets of Langerhans:** Clusters of cells in the pancreas that include the **beta cells,** which make insulin.

Juvenile diabetes: Term once used for **type-I diabetes.**

Ketoacidosis: In diabetes, a dangerous condition caused by very high blood sugars, dehydration and high blood levels of **ketones.**

Ketones: Toxic acids produced by the body when it uses fat instead of glucose for energy.

Ketonuria: Ketones in urine.

Ketosis: Ketones in blood.

Lactose: Sugar found in dairy products.

Lancet: Special needle used for pricking the finger to get a drop of blood; used in self-monitoring of blood glucose.

Latent diabetes: See **impaired glucose tolerance.**

Lente insulin: Intermediate-acting insulin.

Lipid: Fat and/or fatty substance.

Long-acting insulin: Insulin that takes effect slowly and works for a long period of time.

Low-density lipoprotein (LDL): ''Bad'' cholesterol; aids in deposit of fats on artery and cell walls.

Macrovascular: Pertaining to the large blood vessels.

Macula: Area of the retina responsible for sharp, fine vision.

Macular edema: Swelling of the area near the center of retina.

Markers: In diabetes, genetic signposts on a cell that indicate whether diabetes will develop.

Maturity-onset diabetes: Term once used for **type-II diabetes.**

Maturity-onset diabetes of the young: Term sometimes applied for **type-II diabetes** in children and adolescents.

Metabolism: Process of converting food into energy to power the body.

Metformin: Oral hypoglycemic agent; used to lower blood sugar.

Microaneurysm: Small swelling on small blood vessels.

Microvascular: Pertaining to the small blood vessels.

Mixed-split regimen: Diabetes treatment in which mixtures of intermediate-acting insulin and short-acting insulin are given before breakfast and dinner.

Monounsaturated fats: Fats that may protect against vascular disease by lowering LDL cholesterol and raising HDL cholesterol.

Nephropathy: Kidney disease or damage leading to kidney failure.

Neuropathy: Nerve damage resulting in severe pain or loss of feeling.

Non-insulin-dependent diabetes: Term sometimes used for **type-II diabetes.**

Nonketotic coma: Term sometimes used for **hyperosmolar coma.**

Normoglycemia: Normal levels of blood sugar.

NPH insulin: Intermediate-acting insulin.

Onset: When referring to insulin, how quickly insulin takes effect.

Ophthalmologist: Eye doctor, an M.D.

Oral glucose-tolerance test: Series of blood tests used to determine how the body reacts to glucose over a period of several hours.

Oral hypoglycemic agent: Drug used to lower blood sugar in people with **type-II diabetes.** Also called an oral agent.

Oral therapy: Diabetes therapy that uses oral hypoglycemic agents.

Orthostatic hypotension: Sudden drop in blood pressure when a person gets up after reclining.

Pancreas: Gland located behind the stomach that produces insulin, glucagon and other hormones and enzymes.

Peripheral neuropathy: Nerve damage in hands, legs and feet.

Photocoagulation: Use of laser beam to sear leaking blood vessels shut.

Plasma: Blood.

Polydipsia: Long-lasting thirst; symptom of diabetes.

Polyphagia: Unsatisfied hunger; symptom of diabetes.

Polyunsaturated fats: Fatty acids that may reduce LDL cholesterol.

Polyuria: Frequent urination; symptom of diabetes.

Pork-derived insulin: Insulin made from pork pancreas.

Postprandial: After a meal.

Potential abnormality of glucose: Term applied to people who have a close relative with **type-I diabetes** or people with **islet** cell antibodies.

Previous abnormality of glucose tolerance: Term applied to people who have experienced impaired glucose tolerance in the past but have no sign of abnormal glucose metabolism now.

Primary failure: Situation in which an oral hypoglycemic agent fails to lower blood-sugar levels.

Proliferative retinopathy: Advanced disease of retinal blood vessels.

Protein: One of the three basic sources of energy in food; found in fish, meat, eggs and, in lesser amounts, in grains and legumes.

PZI: Protamine zinc insulin; a long-acting insulin.

Reaction denial: Situation in which a person with diabetes does not admit he is having an insulin reaction, usually because blood-glucose levels in the brain are too low.

Rebound: Return to high blood-sugar after levels had been lowered.

Receptors: Structures that serve as gateways to the cell, allowing insulin and other chemicals to enter.

Receptor sites: Places where receptors are located.

Regular insulin: Short-acting insulin.

Renal: Pertaining to kidneys.

Retina: Light-sensing surface on the rear wall of the eye.

Retinopathy: Disease of retinal blood vessels.

Saturated fat: Fat from animal sources that contributes to high cholesterol.

Secondary diabetes: A term used to describe a host of other conditions that can give rise to diabetes. In many such cases, the diabetes is a secondary condition that results from another disease, medication or chemical. Among the causes of secondary diabetes are pancreatic diseases (especially chronic pancreatitis in alcoholics), hormonal abnormalities (including ones that result from the administration of steroids), insulin-receptor disorders, drug- or chemical-induced diabetes and certain genetic syndromes.

Secondary failure: Situation in which an oral hypoglycemic agent that once lowered blood-sugar levels suddenly stops working.

Self-monitoring of blood glucose (SMBG): Technique in which people with diabetes keep track of their day-to-day blood-sugar levels.

Semilente insulin: Short-acting insulin.

Semisynthetic: Term applied to **human insulin** that has been made by chemical modification of **pork-derived insulin.**

Short-acting insulin: Insulin that takes effect quickly.

Simple carbohydrate: Carbohydrate that can be quickly converted to glucose during digestion.

Simple sugar: Simple carbohydrate.

SMBG: Abbreviation for **self-monitoring of blood glucose.**

Soluble fiber: An indigestible material in certain grains, vegetables and fruits that dissolves in water, turning into a thick, gelatinous mass.

Sorbitol: Sweetener used in diet foods; also, a sugar alcohol produced by the body during the conversion of glucose.

Species: Term referring to the source of insulin, whether beef derived, pork derived or synthetically manufactured.

Standard therapy: In diabetes, use of insulin to keep blood-sugar levels within certain target ranges; less stringent than **tight control.**

Stroke: Blockage in the circulation to the brain.

Subcutaneous: Below the skin but above muscle.

Sucrose: Simple sugar.

Sulfonylureas: Class of **oral hypoglycemic agents** or drugs used to lower blood-sugar levels.

Synthetic: Insulin produced in the laboratory through a recombinant DNA process.

Tight control: Type of diabetes therapy that strives for tight control of blood-sugar levels within certain narrow targets. Also known as **intensive therapy.**

Tolazamide: Oral hypoglycemic agent; used to lower blood-sugar levels.

Tolbutamide: Oral hypoglycemic agent; used to lower blood-sugar levels.

Total serum cholesterol: Measurement of overall level of cholesterol in the blood.

Toxemia: The presence of bacterial poison in the bloodstream.

Triglyceride: A compound made up of fatty acid and glycerol; a storage form of fat.

Type-I diabetes: Type of diabetes in which the body loses the capacity to produce insulin. Also called insulin-dependent diabetes or juvenile-onset diabetes.

Type-II diabetes: Type of diabetes in which the body produces some insulin, but that insulin is for some reason ineffective. It usually appears after age 40 and is associated with obesity. Also called non-insulin-dependent diabetes or adult-onset diabetes.

Ultralente insulin: Long-acting insulin.

Ultrasound: Test that uses sound waves to create a picture of organs and structures deep inside the body; used to check the health and development of a fetus and estimate its weight, size and delivery date.

Unsaturated fats: Fatty acids that are liquid at room temperature and that may reduce cholesterol levels.

Vascular: Pertaining to blood vessels.

Vitrectomy: Surgical removal of the **vitreous humor** from the eye.

Vitreous hemorrhage: Major **hemorrhage** in the eye that affects sight.

Vitreous humor: Clear gelatinous material in the center of the eye.

VLDL: Very low-density lipoprotein; a form of fat known as **triglycerides.**

SELECT BIBLIOGRAPHY

American Diabetes Association. *Clinical Practice Recommendations, 1991-1992*. Supplement to *Diabetes Care* 15 (April 1992).

Anderson, James W., M.D., et al. "High-Fiber Diet for Diabetes." *Postgraduate Medicine* 88 (August 1990): 157-68.

Bailey, Clifford J., Ph.D., and Caroline Day, Ph.D. "Traditional Plant Medicines as Treatments for Diabetes." *Diabetes Care* 12 (September 1989): 553-64.

Bankhead, Charles D. "Diabetes Risk Groups Elucidated." *Medical World News* 30 (July 1990): 19-20.

Bernstein, Richard K., M.D. *Diabetes Type II: Living a Long, Healthy Life Through Blood Sugar Normalization*. New York: Prentice Hall, 1990.

Biermann, June, and Barbara Toohey. *The Diabetic's Total Health Book*. New York: Jeremy Tarcher, 1992.

Clements, Bill. "Consumer Interest Pushing Demand for Home Test Kits." *American Medical News* 35 (October 5, 1992).

"Diabetics Tend Not to Feel Hypoglycemia Warnings." *Medical Tribune* 33 (July 9, 1992): 10.

Diabetes Mellitus: Diagnosis and Treatment. 2nd ed. New York: Wiley Medical Publications, 1986.

Dorland's Illustrated Medical Dictionary. 27th ed. Philadelphia: W. B. Saunders, 1988.

Dranov, Paula. *Diabetes: A Random House Personal Medical Handbook*. New York: Random House, 1990.

Dyck, Peter James, M.D. "New Understanding and Treatment of Diabetic Neuropathy." *New England Journal of Medicine* 326 (May 7, 1992): 1287-8.

Early Treatment Diabetic Retinopathy Study Investigators. "Aspirin Effects on Mortality and Morbidity in Patients With Diabetes Mellitus." *Journal of the American Medical Association* 268 (September 9, 1992): 1292-300.

Eisenbarth, George S., M.D., Ph.D. *Type I Diabetes Mellitus: A Chronic and Predictable Autoimmune Disease.* Kalamazoo, Mich.: Upjohn Co., 1989.

Gerich, John E., M.D., and Rose A. Salata, M.D. "Intensive Therapy of Insulin-Dependent Diabetes Mellitus." *Modern Medicine* 57 (February 1989): 88-97.

Golay, A., et al. "High Density Lipoprotein (HDL) Metabolism in Non-Insulin-Dependent Diabetes Mellitus: Measurement of HDL Turnover Using Tritiated HDL." *Journal of Clinical Endocrinology and Metabolism* 65 (1987): 512-8.

Harris, Maureen I., Ph.D., M.P.H., et al. "Onset of NIDDM Occurs at Least 4-7 Years Before Clinical Diagnosis." *Diabetes Care* 15 (July 1992): 815-9.

Helmrich, Susan P., Ph.D., et al. "Physical Activity and Reduced Occurrence of Non-Insulin-Dependent Diabetes Mellitus." *New England Journal of Medicine* 325 (July 18, 1991): 147-52.

Hollander, Priscilla, M.D. "Type II Diabetes." *Postgraduate Medicine* 85 (March 1989): 211-22.

Howard, Barbara V. "Lipoprotein Metabolism in Diabetes Mellitus." *Journal of Lipid Research* 28 (1987): 613-27.

Huse, Daniel M., et al. "The Economic Costs of Non-Insulin-Dependent Diabetes Mellitus." *Journal of the American Medical Association* 262 (November 17, 1989): 2708-13.

Inlander, Charles B., and Paula Brisco. *The Consumer's Guide to Medical Lingo.* Allentown, Pa.: People's Medical Society, 1992.

Jenkins, David, M.D., Ph.D., et al. "Nibbling Versus Gorging: Metabolic Advantages of Increased Meal Frequency." *New England Journal of Medicine* 321 (October 5, 1989): 929-34.

Jovanovic-Peterson, Lois, M.D., et al. *A Touch of Diabetes: A Guide for People Who Have Type II, Non-Insulin-Dependent Diabetes.* Minneapolis: DCI Publishing, 1991.

Karjalainen, J., et al. "A Bovine Albumin Peptide as a Possible Trigger of Insulin-Dependent Diabetes Mellitus." *New England Journal of Medicine* 327 (July 30, 1992): 302-7.

Krall, Leo P., M.D., and Richard S. Beaser, M.D. *Joslin Diabetes Manual.* 12th ed. Philadelphia: Lea & Febiger, 1989.

Lowe, Ernest, and Gary Arsham, M.D., Ph.D. *Diabetes: A Guide to Living Well.* Wayzata, Minn.: Diabetes Center, 1989.

"Male, Female Type II Diabetics Said to Have Similar MI Mortality." *Internal Medicine News & Cardiology News* 25 (August 1, 1992): 38.

McCann, Jean. "Insulin May Delay Diabetes." *Medical Tribune* 33 (August 6, 1992).

Molitch, Mark E., M.D. "Diabetes Mellitus: Control and Complications." *Postgraduate Medicine* 85 (March 1989): 182-94.

Monk, Arlene, R.D., C.D.E., et al. *Managing Type II Diabetes.* Wayzata, Minn.: DCI Publishing, 1988.

Mullin, Lucy, R.N., B.S., C.D.E., and Priscilla Hollander, M.D. "A Practical Guide to Using Insulin." *Postgraduate Medicine* 85 (March 1989): 227-32.

Phillips, Pat. "Hazards of Tight Glucose Control Are Emerging for Type I Diabetes." *Medical World News* 30 (May 28, 1990): 11.

Raskin, Philip, M.D., and Carlos Arauz-Pacheco, M.D. "The Treatment of Diabetic Retinopathy: A View for the Internist." *Annals of Internal Medicine* 116 (April 15, 1992): 226-33.

Reiber, Gayle E., M.P.H., Ph.D., et al. "Risk Factors for Amputation in Patients With Diabetes Mellitus." *Annals of Internal Medicine* 117 (July 15, 1992): 97-105.

Saudek, Christopher D., M.D., et al. "A Preliminary Trial of the Programmable Implantable Medication System for Insulin Delivery." *New England Journal of Medicine* 321 (August 31, 1989): 574-9.

Slom, Celia. "Diet Can Obviate Insulin for Late-Onset Diabetes." *Medical Tribune* 32 (October 31, 1991): 11.

Sorisky, Alexander, M.D., and David C. Robbins, M.D. "Fish Oil and Diabetes: The Net Effect." *Diabetes Care* 12 (April 1989): 302-3.

International Medical News Group. *Special Report on Diabetes.* Supplement to *Internal Medicine News & Cardiology News* 25 (June 1, 1992): 1-22.

Spencer, Martha, M.D. "Type I Diabetes." *Postgraduate Medicine* 85 (March 1989): 201-9.

Strickland, David A. "Self-Monitoring Skills Spotty." *Medical World News* 32 (February 1991): 17.

"Survey Finds Room for Improvement in Diabetes Preventive Care." *Internal Medicine News & Cardiology News* 25 (August 1, 1992): 37.

INDEX

type-II diabetes and, 62-63
Creatinine clearance test, 161-62

D

Dawn phenomenon, 56, 167
Degenerative process, type-II
    diabetes and, 63
Degree, insulin, 43-44, 167
Dehydration, 13-14
    hyperosmolar coma and, 98
    ketoacidosis and, 95-96
Dental care, 155
Diabetes. *See also* Adult-onset
    diabetes, Brittle diabetes,
    Diabetes mellitus, Gestational
    diabetes, Insulin-dependent
    diabetes, Juvenile diabetes,
    Maturity-onset diabetes,
    Maturity-onset diabetes of the
    young, Non-insulin-dependent
    diabetes, Secondary diabetes,
    Type-I diabetes, Type-II diabetes
    aging and, 159
    alcohol and, 25, 77-78, 90, 146
    blood-glucose levels and, 86
    chemical-induced, 25
    complications with, 14-16
        long-term, 88, 99-119
        short-term, 88-99
    cure for, 7
    definition of, 11
    diagnosis of, 16, 27, 30-33
    diet and, 15, 37, 40, 69-73,
        132-50
    drug-induced, 25
    glucose and, 11-13
    incidence of, 15-16
    kinds of, 16, 23
    metabolism and, 11-12, 172
    pregnancy and, 157-58
        (*see also* Gestational diabetes)
    risk factors for, 28-30, 32-33
    screening for, 34
    self-care for, 7-8, 63-64, 121-64
    symptoms of, 11, 13, 27-28
Diabetes mellitus, 11, 167
Diabetic coma. *See* Hyperosmolar
    coma, Ketoacidosis
Dialysis, 109, 167

Diet
    calorie requirements, 143
    cardiovascular disease and, 112-13
    diabetes and, 15, 37, 40, 69-73,
        132-50
    ethnic preferences and, 149
    exchange system, 145
    families and, 134
    fish-oil supplements, 147
    food choices, 133-32
    gestational diabetes and, 27
    glucose intolerance and, 159
    hyperglycemia and, 94
    hypoglycemia and, 50, 90
    information on, 163-64
    insulin and, 31, 44-45, 60, 123,
        134, 141-45, 147
    meal frequency, 143
    nephropathy and, 110
    oral therapy and, 76
    restrictions in, 132-33
    type-I diabetes and, 40, 60
    type-II diabetes and, 21, 37,
        69-73, 83, 167
    vegetarianism, 149
    vitamin supplements, 146-47
Diet therapy, 69-73, 167
Disorientation
    hyperosmolar coma and, 98-99
    ketoacidosis and, 95
Diuretics, blood-glucose levels
    and, 25
Drowsiness
    hyperosmolar coma and, 98-99
    ketoacidosis and, 95, 99
Drug interactions
    insulin and, 51
    oral hypoglycemic agents and, 78
Drugs, blood-glucose levels and, 25
Duration, insulin, 43-44, 167

E

Eating plan. *See* Diet
Elderly, self-care by, 160
Electrocardiogram, 159, 162,
    gestational diabetes and, 159
Environmental factors, type-I
    diabetes and, 32-33
Epinephrine, 92, 168